TOWARD A HEALTHY SOCIETY

This book offers new ideas for aligning the American health care system to optimize health for everyone. Bridging real-world examples and innovative strategies, it leverages a patient-centric framework to explore health care lifecycles and identify primary groups in its ecosystem. The chapters explore critical topics from a comparative global perspective, including the role of government in driving access, the private sector's contribution to quality, and the value of integrating social determinants in policy to achieve health equity. By advocating for public–private collaboration, this work presents actionable solutions to challenges facing the country's modern health care system such as resource allocation and long wait times. Designed for health care professionals, policymakers, and advocates, it highlights the need for bipartisan approaches, cutting-edge patient care models, and the integration of empathy and culture in health care delivery. Addressing affordability, equity, and inclusivity, this book equips readers with a roadmap for reimagining health care systems that truly serve everyone.

GREGORY J. PRIVITERA is a Professor in Psychology at St. Bonaventure University, where he is a recipient of its highest teaching honor and its highest honor for research and scholarship. He is a three-time national award-winning author, and best-selling author. His widely recognized research bridges knowledge creation across the health and health care policy space.

JAMES J. GILLESPIE is an Assistant Professor in Business and Management at Saint Mary's College, a Senior Advisor at McKinsey & Company, and a Senior Advisor at Stanford School of Medicine. His research focuses on the management, policy, and strategic dimensions of the health care sector. He has been published in many leading academic and practitioner journals.

TOWARD A HEALTHY SOCIETY

Comparative Perspectives on American Health Care Policy

GREGORY J. PRIVITERA
St. Bonaventure University, New York

JAMES J. GILLESPIE
Saint Mary's College, Indiana

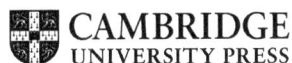

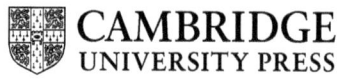

Shaftesbury Road, Cambridge CB2 8EA, United Kingdom

One Liberty Plaza, 20th Floor, New York, NY 10006, USA

477 Williamstown Road, Port Melbourne, VIC 3207, Australia

314–321, 3rd Floor, Plot 3, Splendor Forum, Jasola District Centre, New Delhi – 110025, India

103 Penang Road, #05–06/07, Visioncrest Commercial, Singapore 238467

Cambridge University Press is part of Cambridge University Press & Assessment, a department of the University of Cambridge.

We share the University's mission to contribute to society through the pursuit of education, learning and research at the highest international levels of excellence.

www.cambridge.org
Information on this title: www.cambridge.org/9781009625869

DOI: 10.1017/9781009625821

© Gregory J. Privitera and James J. Gillespie 2025

This publication is in copyright. Subject to statutory exception and to the provisions of relevant collective licensing agreements, no reproduction of any part may take place without the written permission of Cambridge University Press & Assessment.

When citing this work, please include a reference to the DOI 10.1017/9781009625821

First published 2025

Cover image: *Healthy Heart*. Carol Yepes via Getty Images.

A catalogue record for this publication is available from the British Library

A Cataloging-in-Publication data record for this book is available from the Library of Congress

ISBN 978-1-009-62586-9 Hardback
ISBN 978-1-009-62585-2 Paperback

Cambridge University Press & Assessment has no responsibility for the persistence or accuracy of URLs for external or third-party internet websites referred to in this publication and does not guarantee that any content on such websites is, or will remain, accurate or appropriate.

For EU product safety concerns, contact us at Calle de José Abascal, 56, 1°, 28003 Madrid, Spain, or email eugpsr@cambridge.org

It is with a heavy heart, sincere gratitude, and love that this book is dedicated to Dr. Chanel Simone Freeman, a practitioner who embraced life with a passion and purpose that left a lasting impact on everyone who knew her.

From Dr. Privitera: *Dr. Chanel Freeman was one of those rare students whose light left an eternal imprint on everyone she encountered – including me. As her professor early in our careers, I quickly realized that her brilliance, resilience, and spirit were a gift to our campus and to my own growth as an educator. Her life reflected the very spirit of this book – one that calls for empathy, advocacy, and collaboration to innovate a more inclusive, holistic health care future for us all. May this dedication be a testimony to the enduring impact one soul can have on many, simply by embodying love, courage, and purpose.*

From Mom and family: *Chanel Simone Freeman was born on August 22, 1991, in the Bronx, NY, and from the start, she was a force of purpose and passion. If told she couldn't do something, Chanel would work twice as hard to prove she could. That fierce determination led her to accomplish more in thirty-one years than many do in a lifetime.*
After graduating from Bronx Law and Government High School, Chanel earned a BA in psychology from St. Bonaventure University in 2013. Inspired to help others

through health care, she went on to achieve her BSN, MSN, and ultimately her Doctor of Nursing Practice from Pace University in 2022. Her journey included internships and clinical service, including her dream job as an RN for Hospital Special Surgery and Regional Manager for CVS Mini Clinic – always serving with excellence and empathy. Chanel built an impressive career at a young age, receiving many honors and impacting everyone she met along the way – her impact can still be felt among those who knew her.

Chanel was known for "understanding the assignment." She excelled academically, but more importantly, she embodied joy, integrity, and purpose in every space she entered. She traveled widely, lived boldly, and walked in unwavering faith. As a lifelong member of Greater Zion Hill Baptist Church of Harlem, she served and gave with a full heart.

She embraced every challenge with brilliance and embodied the essence of Black Girl Excellence. *Chanel's life was a testament to what is possible when grace, strength, and faith work together.*

Gone too soon – but never forgotten. Mommy Chanel's favorite charity was her church, Greater Zion Hill Baptist Church. If interested, please consider donating @givelify https://giv.li/5tfcry and add a note that your gift is "In Honor of Dr. Chanel S. Freeman."

Contents

List of Figures	*page* x
List of Tables	xi
Preface	xiii
About the Authors	xvii
Acknowledgements	xviii

1		Moving toward a Healthy Society	1
	1.1	Equity and Justice in Health Care	3
	1.2	Four Major Models for Systems of Health Care	4
	1.3	An Optimal Health Care System: Measuring Quality, Access, and Cost	8
	1.4	The 6 Ps Framework for Health Care	12
	1.5	Across the Pond: How Are Health and Diversity Related?	19
	1.6	Moving toward a Healthy Society	22
		Chapter Summary	23
2		Paying the Most, Getting the Least	24
	2.1	Comparative Analysis of the US Health Care System	25
	2.2	US Spending on Health Care: Price per Unit versus Total Utilization	27
	2.3	Accessibility and Affordability	29
	2.4	Equity and Disparities	30
	2.5	Not All Gloom and Doom: Areas Where the United States Excels	32
	2.6	Across the Pond: Health Care Insurance Uncovered, Nonuniversal	34
	2.7	Disparities in US Health Care: The Need for Positive Change	35
		Chapter Summary	37
3		Government Drives Access	38
	3.1	Across the Pond: Aligning Incentives in Health Care	39
	3.2	Cost as a Primary Barrier	42
	3.3	Access as a Secondary Barrier	44
	3.4	Nonhealth Determinants of Health	46
	3.5	Mobile Clinics, School-Based Health Centers, and Telehealth	48
	3.6	Universal Health Care and Other Government Solutions	50
		Chapter Summary	52

Contents

4 Private Industry as a Partner in Health Care — 53
 4.1 Public–Private Partnerships — 54
 4.2 Leveraging the Private Sector in Health Care — 57
 4.3 Advantages and Disadvantages of the Public and Private Sector — 59
 4.4 Mixed Systems in US Health Care — 61
 4.5 Across the Pond: The Complexity of US Health Care — 63
 4.6 The Role of Government with Private-Sector Providers — 65
 Chapter Summary — 67

5 Health Needs to Be about People, Not Politics — 69
 5.1 Across the Pond: The Basis for Polarization — 70
 5.2 Increasing Partisanship and Polarization — 72
 5.3 Polarization Hurts Patient Health and Policymaking — 76
 5.4 Reducing Polarization – Generally — 78
 5.5 Reducing Polarization – Specific Examples — 80
 5.6 Data and Technology as Enablers of Depolarization — 83
 Chapter Summary — 86

6 The Affordable Care Act: Why Is It So Unaffordable? — 87
 6.1 ACA Beginnings, Launch, Goals, and Achievements — 88
 6.2 Costs for Government, Employers, and Patients under ACA — 90
 6.3 Externalities, Incentives, and Outcomes for Patients under ACA — 93
 6.4 Across the Pond: Externalities and Incentives for Providers and Payers — 96
 6.5 Artificial Intelligence as a Tool for Shaping Health Care Policy — 97
 Chapter Summary — 100

7 The Health Care Debate: Is It Too Focused on Insurance? — 101
 7.1 Health Equity and the Social Determinants of Health — 102
 7.2 The Social Determinants and Health Policy — 105
 7.3 Thinking beyond the Point of Care — 107
 7.4 Examples of Policy in the United States and Abroad — 109
 7.5 Across the Pond: What Is Medicine? — 114
 Chapter Summary — 116

8 Health Equity: Is It Even Possible? — 117
 8.1 Barriers to Health Equity — 118
 8.2 The Principle of *Meeting People Where They Are* — 123
 8.3 Policy Considerations for Closing Health Disparity Gaps — 124
 8.4 Strategies for Health Policy Change — 125
 8.5 Across the Pond: Addressing Social Determinants of Health — 131
 Chapter Summary — 132

9 Moving toward More Inclusive Health Care Policy — 134
 9.1 The Whole Being Model: A Holistic Approach — 135
 9.2 Steps toward Inclusive Health Care Policy — 138
 9.3 Closing Health Disparity Gaps: Key Themes — 146

9.4	Humanizing Patients in the Health Care Ecosystem	147
9.5	Across the Pond: The Whole Being Model in Policy	149
	Chapter Summary	151

10 Expanding the Role of Patients in Health Care   152

10.1	Patient-Centric Care: Community-Engaged Health Care	153
10.2	Expanding the Role of Providers: Lessons Learned from the Pandemic	155
10.3	Aligning the Interests of HCOs and Community Leaders	157
10.4	Exploring Innovation for Financial Incentive Models	160
10.5	Across the Pond: Putting People over Politics	163
	Chapter Summary	165

Glossary   166
Bibliography   173
Index   189

Figures

1.1	Factors that affect the health of a society	page 2
1.2	The Donabedian model for measuring health care quality	9
1.3	The 6 Ps pentagonal framework for health care	12
2.1	Life expectancy and expenditure	26
2.2	People of color more likely to die	31
2.3	Health disparities	31
3.1	Misaligned incentives in US health care	40
5.1	Pathway to and from polarization in US health care policymaking	75
6.1	Employer premiums, deductibles, and wages since 2010	92
6.2	Life expectancy	95
7.1	The CSDH conceptual framework for the social determinants of health	104
7.2	The CSDH conceptual framework for addressing health inequities	106
8.1	Leveraging healthy people to advance health equity	119
8.2	Six key policy differences between the ACA and the AHCA	127
9.1	The whole being model in health care: patient, person, and consumer – connected to fourteen key steps needed in the United States to move toward a more inclusive health care policy	136
10.1	Conceptual model to advance health equity through transformed systems for health	154
10.2	Personalizing rewards using good target incentives for patients to reach health goals	162

Tables

1.1	Four major models for health care systems	*page* 5
1.2	Measuring health care costs	10
1.3	The score and ranking for health and ethnic diversity of a nation	21

Preface

Framing an Equitable Future for Health Care

In this book, we frame an equitable future for health care by focusing on what we refer to as the *axes of the US health care debate*: government and equity. We address government in terms of their involvement in health care, with the perspective that the data itself supports the need for government involvement in health care to ensure *access* for all. We address equity by asking, "Is the health care debate too focused on insurance for all?" While access to health care is essential, factors outside the health care system account for about 80 percent of the variability in quality-of-life and length-of-life measures. We therefore posit that to achieve health equity, we must go further than simply insuring everyone, by integrating the social determinants of health (SDOH) into health care policy as well. Hence, this text provides a focused, data-driven discussion about two of the most critical, yet related, policy constraints in the US health care debate: one that is widely debated (federal government involvement), and one that is, by comparison, scarcely debated (inclusion of social determinants *in health care policy*).

A major point of contention in the US health care policy debate is federal government involvement. In this book, we follow the data, both nationally and internationally, to explore the utility of federal governments' role in health care. What are their strengths and their weaknesses? How can this inform the ability of the federal government to successfully be involved in US health care? We further explore the need to prioritize SDOH in health care policy. Again, we follow the data, nationally and internationally, to determine how such prioritization can meaningfully close health disparities. In this way, the book is focused on a conversation that converges the value of health care access with *meeting people where they are*, to optimize access and equity within a health care system. Overall, this book engages in an inclusive conversation around health care policy.

In Chapter 1, we use the 6 Ps model for health care, which treats patients as the foundation of any health care system. The system exists to serve them and, by extension, their health. An optimal health care system optimizes the health for all members in a population. The metrics for an optimal system are also introduced as ensuring that all people have *access* to *quality* care they can *afford* (costs). We further operationalize how the metrics for an optimal health care system translate to achieving its goal of optimizing the health of all the people it serves.

In this book, we move from a discussion on the structure of health care to a conversation around equity in care. We begin by asking questions. What are the health care needs of a diverse nation (Chapter 2)? What are the advantages and cautions for federal government involvement in health care (Chapter 3)? A key theme in the early chapters is the value of having a universal health care *option*. Particularly, we focus on the key metric of *access* to health care, with examples provided to showcase the value of a universal health care option as a way of closing health equity gaps by ensuring that all members in a society can utilize health care.

We transition to a broader discussion to align bipartisan perspectives in health care policy. In Chapter 4, we focus on the key metric of *quality* of health care by exploring the potential synergies between private industry and public health care. In Chapters 5 and 6, we expand the conversation further by assessing not only the utility of health care policy in the United States but also by aligning policy with the perspective that health is about people, not politics. We provide context for how health care became such a political issue (e.g., the rollout of Affordable Care Act [ACA]; ideological differences between parties), and the need to align solutions across party lines in the United States. A broader theme that extends throughout this book is the need to prioritize patients in health care solutions.

Beginning in Chapter 7, we shift to an emphasis on health equity. We explore the health care debate's narrow focus on insurance as a pathway to accessibility, arguing that while necessary, it is insufficient for achieving health equity. True health equity extends beyond the point of care to address SDOH – the lived environments and socioeconomic factors that shape health outcomes. We propose that recognizing SDOH as "medicine" could redefine health care policy, fostering equity through holistic, patient-centered, and socially adaptive approaches.

As the book progresses, we explore the feasibility of health equity in the United States (Chapter 8), and we introduce the whole being model as a framework for inclusive health care, emphasizing the interplay between an individual's roles as a patient, consumer, and person (Chapter 9).

Strategies for bipartisan solutions and public–private partnerships are presented as pathways to sustainable, inclusive health policies that prioritize equity beyond the point of care. We posit that by humanizing patients and prioritizing cultural competence, we can readily achieve inclusive health care policy.

In the closing chapter, we bring the themes of the book to a meaningful conclusion by focusing on the evolving roles of patients and providers in fostering a more inclusive and equitable health care system. The conclusion appeals to collaborative efforts among stakeholders – the 6 Ps (patients, policy makers, pharmacies, pharmaceuticals, payers, and providers) – to establish patient-centered health care policies that promote a vision for an inclusive health care future.

The overall perspective of this book is that having access to care allows us to *be healthy*; meeting people where they are, to address SDOH as an integrated part of policy, allows us to *live healthy*. Optimizing the health of all people – which extends beyond the health care system itself – must therefore be the primary goal of all stakeholders. To the extent that we agree on this, bipartisan solutions can be readily achieved by aligning interests across the 6 Ps (i.e., the stakeholders) in the health care system.

Thank you for choosing *Toward a Healthy Society*. We hope it achieves its aims, described here, to foster a framework of understanding health care in a way that can inspire conversation over debate and put people over politics.

About the Authors

GREGORY J. PRIVITERA is a professor of psychology at St. Bonaventure University, where he is a recipient of their highest teaching honor and their highest honor for scholarship. He also works in industry as Chief Data and Analytics Officer for Umoja Health, where he supports cross-functional initiatives and assessment of programs aimed at closing health disparities in underserved communities. He received his PhD at the State University of New York at Buffalo, and completed his postdoctoral work at Arizona State University. Dr. Privitera is a three-time national-award-winning author of texts across the statistics and methodology space. His research in the health and health policy space is highly cited, and has produced nearly four dozen peer-reviewed papers with his work being nationally recognized by the American Psychological Association. Dr. Privitera is a veteran of the United States Marine Corps (Semper Fi!), is an identical twin, and is married with four children: two daughters, Grace Ann and Charlotte Jane, and two sons, Aiden Andrew and Luca James.

JAMES J. GILLESPIE is a faculty member in business and management at Saint Mary's College, Notre Dame, IN, USA. He focuses on research, teaching, and consulting in the management, operational, and strategic dimensions of the health care and life sciences sectors. James also is a senior advisor at McKinsey & Company and a senior advisor at Stanford University School of Medicine. He was previously a research affiliate at the Yale University School of Medicine. James is President and Co-Founder of the Center for Health Care Innovation, an education and research institution focused on health equity. He has published in many leading academic and industry journals. He is the co-author of *Patient-Centric Analytics in Health Care: Driving Value in Clinical Settings and Psychological Practice* by Rowman & Littlefield. His education includes Northwestern University Kellogg School (PhD and MS), Harvard University Law School (JD), Princeton University (MPA), Massachusetts Institute of Technology (BS), and Carnegie Mellon University. He is honored to have served in the United States Army Reserve.

Acknowledgements

We would like to convey a special thanks to Brian Talant for his invaluable copyediting and manuscript preparation support throughout the process of developing this book.

From Dr. Privitera: To my sons, Aiden Andrew and Luca James, and my daughters, Grace Ann and Charlotte Jane – every moment I am with you is the greatest moment of my life. I often teach that confidence in the absence of humility is arrogance. It is in those moments that I share with my children that I find my humility each day. May this work be a humble step toward a future for an inclusive health care future for all.

From Dr. Gillespie: To frontline health care workers.

CHAPTER 1

Moving toward a Healthy Society

Insights

- Social determinants drive health outcomes, with about 80 percent of quality of life and length of life being influenced by factors outside the health care system.
- Addressing systemic inequalities (justice) offers longer-term solutions, rather than focusing solely on equality or equity.
- US health care combines four health care models into one, creating a complex and fragmented system.
- Aligning interests across the 6 Ps is essential for effective, patient-centered health care reform.
- Greater racial diversity correlates with lower health rankings, highlighting the need for tailored, inclusive policies.

When we think of health care policy, more often than not, we are discussing how to ensure all people can see their doctor and get the care they need. While a doctor's office may often be at the forefront of where health care occurs, it is *how* we live that has the greatest effect on our health. From the moment we take our first breath to our last, every moment in between affects our health. Having access to quality health care is the low-hanging fruit; it's the very least a nation can achieve. Why? Because most predictors of our quality of life and length of life occur outside a health care system. Factors such as economic and family stability, community and social factors, the neighborhood and built food environments within which we live, the quality of our work and workplace, and the access and quality of our educational system all have a substantial impact on our quality of life and length of life. It is common sense for health care policy, then, to be inclusive of more than just getting people to a doctor. After all, health care encompasses all the spaces within which we live.

There are approximately 8,765 hours in a year, and doctors generally ask for only one of those hours annually. Even then, only about 83 percent of adults will visit a doctor or other health care professional in a given year.[1] Broadly speaking, the challenges for patient care in clinical settings have two constraints: those for the primary care physicians and those for the patients. For primary care physicians, the constraint is largely having sufficient time to provide adequate care. After all, they typically only see a patient once a year unless there is an ailment or pathology that requires more time. For patients, the constraint is largely that of adherence. After all, nearly all year long, they are anywhere but in a primary care physician's office.

Consider, for example, that two people have access to the same doctor. Suppose they are both diagnosed as prediabetic and go home with a prescription to eat healthier and exercise more. They have access to the same doctor, but is that enough? Notably, as illustrated in Figure 1.1,

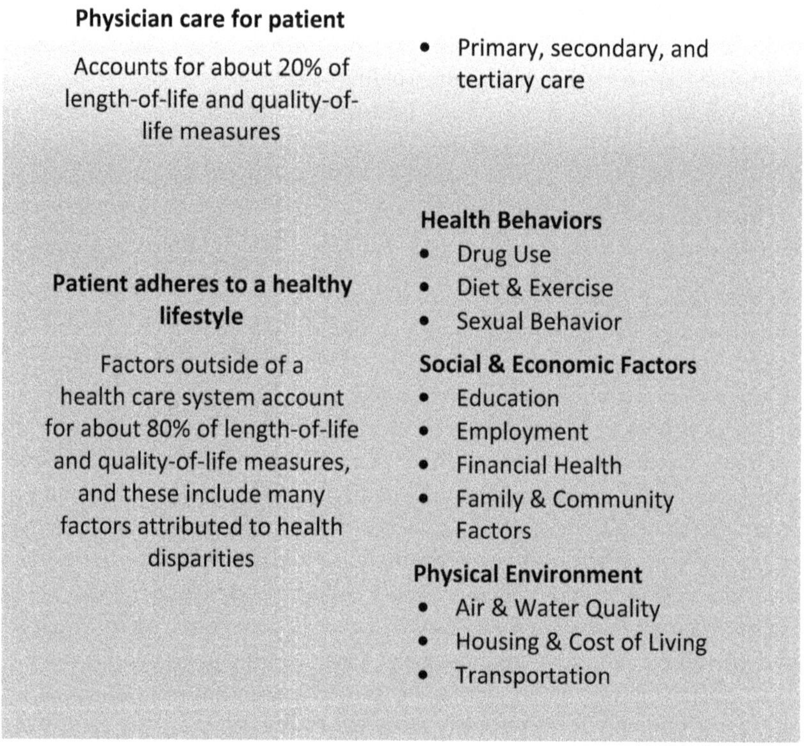

Physician care for patient	
Accounts for about 20% of length-of-life and quality-of-life measures	• Primary, secondary, and tertiary care
Patient adheres to a healthy lifestyle	**Health Behaviors** • Drug Use • Diet & Exercise • Sexual Behavior
Factors outside of a health care system account for about 80% of length-of-life and quality-of-life measures, and these include many factors attributed to health disparities	**Social & Economic Factors** • Education • Employment • Financial Health • Family & Community Factors **Physical Environment** • Air & Water Quality • Housing & Cost of Living • Transportation

Figure 1.1 Factors that affect the health of a society

[1] Centers for Disease Control and Prevention (CDC), "Ambulatory Care Use."

factors outside a health care system – those related to the backdrop of *how we live* – account for about 80 percent of length-of-life and quality-of-life outcomes, and these include many factors attributed to health disparities. Continuing with our example, if one person lives in a poorer environment that is less safe, less walkable, and further from a grocery store, with poorer transportation, they will have a more difficult time following the prescription to eat healthier and exercise more. In other words, despite having access to the same doctor, the health disparities that drive inequity between these two individuals still persist.

1.1 Equity and Justice in Health Care

Equity, equality, and justice are often used in discussions about fairness, especially in the context of health care systems. A common strategy to address inequality involves efforts to achieve equality or equity. However, these efforts alone are often insufficient to address inequality in the long term. Rather, efforts toward justice as a means of addressing inequality tend to be better suited to achieve long-term success because in doing so, health disparities can be closed by addressing the underlying causes of inequalities in the system itself. In health care, there is therefore a need to think beyond equality and equity to seek health justice.

To illustrate the need for health justice, let's revisit our example for two people with access to the same doctor and both are diagnosed as prediabetic. They go home with a prescription to eat healthier and exercise more. Let's consider eating healthier in terms of access to getting groceries. When there is inequality, one person has easier access to a grocery store than the other.

- To achieve **equality**, we can distribute resources evenly to all people in the same way. For example, we could give each person a grocery allowance of $100 per month. However, recall that one person lives further from a grocery store and has poorer transportation options, making it more difficult for them to get to a grocery store to spend those dollars. Inequalities that could be addressed still exist.
- To achieve **equity**, we could customize the resources provided to meet the unique needs of each individual. For example, we could give each person a grocery allowance, but give the person from the poorer environment more money to spend on the card. However, this does not address the underlying causes of the inequality in that one person

still lives further from a grocery store, with poorer transportation. Inequalities that could be addressed still exist.
- To achieve **justice**, we could fix the system to offer equal access to both the resources and the opportunities. For example, the first person can receive the $100 per month grocery allowance, which would suffice for their needs. The person living in the poorer environment can receive the card plus a door-drop service to deliver groceries straight to their door, thereby alleviating the underlying cause of the inequality – their inability to get to a grocery store. In the effort to close health disparities, achieving justice allowed for longer-term success.

Certainly, health care is a complex problem to solve, but it is solvable. For example, we witnessed equity in action with the distribution of vaccines during the COVID-19 pandemic. To directly and quickly reach all communities, including those that were underserved or high-risk, the US federal government created programs such as the Federal Retail Pharmacy Program, the Health Center COVID-19 Vaccine Program, Rural Health Clinic COVID-19 programs, tribal health programs, and Urban Indian Organizations, all of which helped to realize a record distribution of vaccines across the country.[2]

In this book, we evaluate the American health care system and explore how the top health care countries in the world can help to inform US health care policy, in part, to alleviate inequalities in the system. To begin, first we briefly introduce the four major models for health care systems, and then we will introduce the landscape of American health care using the 6 Ps framework, developed by the authors of this text.[3]

1.2 Four Major Models for Systems of Health Care

There are generally four major health care models that are utilized in different ways globally: the Beveridge model, the Bismarck model, the National Health Insurance Model, and the out-of-pocket model. To some extent, most countries typically do not choose one or the other model. Instead, most tend to structure their health care system by featuring one or more of these major models.[4] Each major model for a health care system is summarized in Table 1.1 and described in this section.

---

[2] U.S. Department of Health and Human Services (HHS), "COVID-19 Vaccines."
[3] Gillespie and Privitera, *Patient-Centric Analytics*.   [4] Chung, "Healthcare Reform."

1.2 Four Major Models for Systems of Health Care

Table 1.1 *Four major models for health care systems*

Models for health care	Description	Examples	Key strength/limitation
Beveridge model	A system in which the government acts as the single-payer, providing health care coverage for all citizens through income tax payments	United Kingdom, Spain, New Zealand, Cuba	Strength: Costs can be kept low and benefits can be standardized across the country Limitation: Overutilization of the system due to everyone being guaranteed access to health services may lead to increasing costs
Bismarck model	Characterized by mandatory employer and employee contributions through payroll deductions to fund health insurance plans	Germany, Belgium, Japan, Switzerland	Strength: Government can implement control over prices for health services because the insurers do not make a profit Limitation: Identifying how to care for those who are unable to work or those who may not be able to afford contributions
National Health Insurance Model	Combines aspects of the Beveridge and Bismarck models, with the government acting as a single-payer while providers remain private	Canada, Taiwan, South Korea	Strength: This system covers most procedures regardless of income level and can reduce the costs of health insurance Limitation: Overutilization of health resources in nonurgent situations and long waiting lists for patients to see a physician
Out-of-pocket model	Represents the absence of a formalized health care system in which individuals must pay for their own medical expenses out of pocket	India, China, Africa, South America	Strength: Those who have the ability to pay can do so through insurance options Limitation: Disparities in wealth lead to disparities in health outcomes because the poor are unable to afford health care

Note: The United States is a fragmented health system that incorporates aspects of all four models.

The Beveridge Model

The **Beveridge model**, first developed by Sir William Beveridge in the United Kingdom in 1948, is a system in which the government acts as the single-payer, providing health care coverage for all citizens through income tax payments. This system is often simply called a *single-payer system*. In the United States, the Veterans Health Administration operates under the Beveridge model and is generally considered a socialized system, employing government-funded and government-managed care. Similarly, the Medicare program operates partly under the Beveridge model, with the government acting as a single-payer of health services for citizens aged sixty-five or older.

This system is often centralized through a national health service. The government acts as the single-payer, thereby eliminating market competition and volatility that generally work to keep prices low. Using income taxes to fund health care allows for patient care to be free at the point of service with the patient not having to pay any out-of-pocket fees because of their contribution through taxes. Each citizen is guaranteed by the government the same universal access to care, with a central tenet of this model being that *health is a human right*.

The Bismarck Model

The **Bismarck model**, created near the end of the nineteenth century by Otto von Bismarck, is characterized by mandatory employer and employee contributions through payroll deductions to fund health insurance plans. In the United States, a significant portion of the population receives health coverage through employer-sponsored insurance plans, which, at first glance, seems like an application of the Bismarck model. However, the Bismarck model works under the assumption that the insurers are nonprofit. This is not the case in the United States, with insurers operating for-profit, thereby diverging somewhat from the Bismarck model.

This system is a more decentralized form of health care. Health providers are generally private institutions, though the insurers are considered public. In some countries, there is a single insurer (e.g., France and Korea); others may have multiple, competing insurers (e.g., Germany and the Czech Republic); still others may have multiple, noncompeting insurers (e.g., Japan). Because the insurers do not make a profit, this allows the government to implement control over prices for health services.

The National Health Insurance Model

The **National Health Insurance Model** combines aspects of the Beveridge and Bismarck models, with the government acting as a single-payer while providers remain private. In the United States, the Medicare program partly incorporates elements of this model as well, with the government financing health care costs through payroll taxes and premiums, but the delivery of care remains in the hands of private providers rather than a centralized system. Using this system, there are generally fewer financial barriers to care and patients are usually able to choose their health care providers. Public insurance and private practice are balanced as well, thereby allowing hospitals to be independent while also reducing complications with insurance policies.

The Out-of-Pocket Model

The **out-of-pocket model** represents the absence of a formalized health care system in which individuals must pay for their own medical expenses out of pocket. In the United States, a portion of the population remains uninsured and must therefore pay for health care costs out of pocket, which is similar to this model. The out-of-pocket model often results in significant health disparities in which those least capable of paying for their care (i.e., the uninsured) are asked to pay the most; meanwhile, the wealthy can afford medical care through insurance options that reduce their financial burden to access health care. Using this system, disparities in wealth lead to disparities in health outcomes. Less developed nations have too few resources, leaving patients to pay for their health care out of pocket. Unfortunately, this system is common in most nations, with only the wealthiest countries having robust health care systems.

The United States stands out as the only industrialized nation that lacks a uniform, universal health care system for its entire population. Instead, the United States employs a fragmented approach, incorporating aspects of all four models (Beveridge, Bismarck, National Health Insurance, and out-of-pocket) for different segments of the population. This fragmentation results in a complex and multifaceted health care system that differs from most other countries, which typically adopt a single or hybrid model uniformly across their populations. The fragmented nature of US health care also means that there are many "players" in this system, with varying interests that are not always aligned to optimize patient health. In the next section, we use the 6 Ps framework for US health care[5] to take a closer look at the "players" in this system, to find out who they are, and the types of questions they ask.

1.3 An Optimal Health Care System: Measuring Quality, Access, and Cost

Using the 6 Ps model of health care, patients are regarded as the foundation of any health care system. The system exists to serve them and, by extension, their health. An optimal health care system therefore optimizes the health for all members of its population. Using the 6 Ps model, three core metrics are used to measure the strength of health care policy in terms of the extent to which it ensures that all people have *access* to *quality* care that they can afford (*costs*). Moving toward a healthy society – the title of this book – reflects a holistic perspective in which there is a continuous pursuit to optimize each metric (quality, access, and cost) for a population. Each metric is critical to serving the health care needs of a nation, and is therefore summarized here before introducing the 6 Ps framework.

Quality is a measure of the excellence of care. While countries use various approaches to measure the quality of health care, one widely utilized approach is the **Donabedian model**, which was developed by Avedis Donabedian, who is widely regarded as the father of modern health care quality management. Using this model, summarized in Figure 1.2, health care quality measures are classified into three categories: structure, process, and outcome.[6] As represented using arrows, the structure of health care using this model has influence on the processes of care, which, in turn, can influence the effect of care on health status.

Access is the ease with which patients can utilize care in the system; the system is most accessible when all patients can seamlessly utilize it for care. There are many ways in which access can be measured. The first is at a national level using the **Healthcare Access and Quality (HAQ) Index**, which is a comprehensive measure used to evaluate and compare the quality of national health care access.[7] This index is measured on a scale from 0 (least accessible) to 100 (most accessible), based on death rates from

---

[5] Gillespie and Privitera, *Patient-Centric Analytics*.
[6] Donabedian, "Evaluating the Quality of Medical Care."
[7] Younas et al., "Sociocultural and Patient-Healthcare."

1.3 Measuring Health Care Quality, Access, and Cost

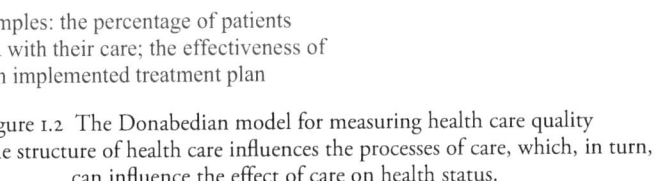

Structure
assesses features of a health care organization to include the setting, policies, funds and assets, and resources available to providers of care that are relevant to their capacity to provide good health care

Examples: the ratio of providers to patients; the efficiency of an emergency room

Process
assesses steps that should be followed to provide good care such that the process, if executed well, will increase the likelihood of achieving a desired outcome

Examples: the utility of diagnostic procedures; the percentage of people receiving necessary preventive services

Outcome
assesses the health status of a patient, or their change in health status (desirable or adverse), resulting from receiving care

Examples: the percentage of patients satisfied with their care; the effectiveness of an implemented treatment plan

Quality
a measure of the excellence of care

Figure 1.2 The Donabedian model for measuring health care quality
Note: The structure of health care influences the processes of care, which, in turn, can influence the effect of care on health status.

32 causes of death that could be avoided with proper medical care. The HAQ Index is a useful tool for monitoring national levels of health care access and quality.[8]

Other methods of measuring access to health care include: (i) availability of health care services, (ii) geographical accessibility of care, (iii) equity in health care access, and (iv) the efficiency and timeliness of health care access. The availability of health care services is most often measured by calculating the number of hospitals or health facilities per population. The geographical accessibility of care is often measured by assessing the travel time or distance to reach the nearest health care facility or needed services. Equity in health care access is crucial for identifying health disparities and

---

[8] GBD 2019 Collaborators, "Assessing Performance."

is a measure of health care access across different demographic groups, such as those based on income levels, race, ethnicity, sex, geographic location, or other socioeconomic and sociodemographic factors. Countries also measure the efficiency and timeliness of health care access, such as waiting times for appointments or procedures, and the ability of the health care system to provide care without harmful delays. Efficient health care systems maximize the benefits of available resources while avoiding risks and waste.[9]

The *costs* of health care tend to be the trickiest metric to solve. Costs reflect the expenditures required to make the system efficient in terms of the time, money, and resources needed to provide care for a population. Assessing costs is relatively challenging because there are many methods that can be considered. Each method of measuring costs in health care is summarized in Table 1.2. Different methods allow for different ways of gaining insights into how much money is being spent and the extent to which spending is efficient.

Table 1.2 *Measuring health care costs*

Method of measuring health care spending	What does it measure?	What information does it convey?
National Health Expenditure as a share of gross domestic product (GDP)	Measures health care costs in the United States with the National Health Expenditure as a share of GDP	It provides a comprehensive overview of how much the nation allocates to health care relative to its overall economic output
Per capita health spending	Measures per capita health spending in the United States	It offers insights into individual health care needs and how they change over time, providing a clear picture of the financial burden that health care puts on the average American
Personal Health Care Expenditures	Encompasses various categories of health care spending, including hospital care, physician and clinical services, prescription drugs, and other personal health care costs	It represents a substantial portion of the total health care costs in the United States, accounting for about 85 percent of National Health Expenditures

[9] World Health Organization, "Quality of Care."

Table 1.2 (cont.)

Method of measuring health care spending	What does it measure?	What information does it convey?
Out-of-pocket costs	Encompasses direct payments made by individuals for health care services, excluding insurance premiums	The impact of out-of-pocket costs on overall health care expenses is influenced by factors such as insurance coverage, health status, and the types of medical services received
Health Insurance Expenditures	Encompasses public and private health insurance spending to include Medicare and Medicaid spending	It highlights the significant role that both private and public insurance play in overall health care costs
Health Care Price Indices	Price indices include: Consumer Price Index, which measures changes in the prices paid by urban consumers for medical care commodities and services, the Producer Price Index, which reflects inflation from the providers' perspective, focusing on actual transaction prices, and Personal Consumption Expenditures, which tracks changes in prices paid on behalf of consumers, including payments by employers, private insurers, and government programs	These indices assess changes in health care costs over time
Sector-specific expenditures	Breaks down expenditures into specific sectors	Sector-specific measures provide detailed insights into which areas of health care are experiencing the most substantial cost increases
Public vs. private spending	Distinguishes between public and private spending	It helps in understanding the distribution of health care costs across different sectors of society and the economy

1.4 The 6 Ps Framework for Health Care

The health care landscape in the United States is multitiered and not always aligned toward optimizing patient health, which creates its own challenges in developing a uniform, universal health care system for an entire population. Figure 1.3 identifies the **6 Ps pentagonal framework for health care**[10] with examples for the industries in each *P* (i.e., for each health care sector or entity) provided. The 6 Ps identified in Figure 1.3 are as follows:

- Patients
- Policy makers

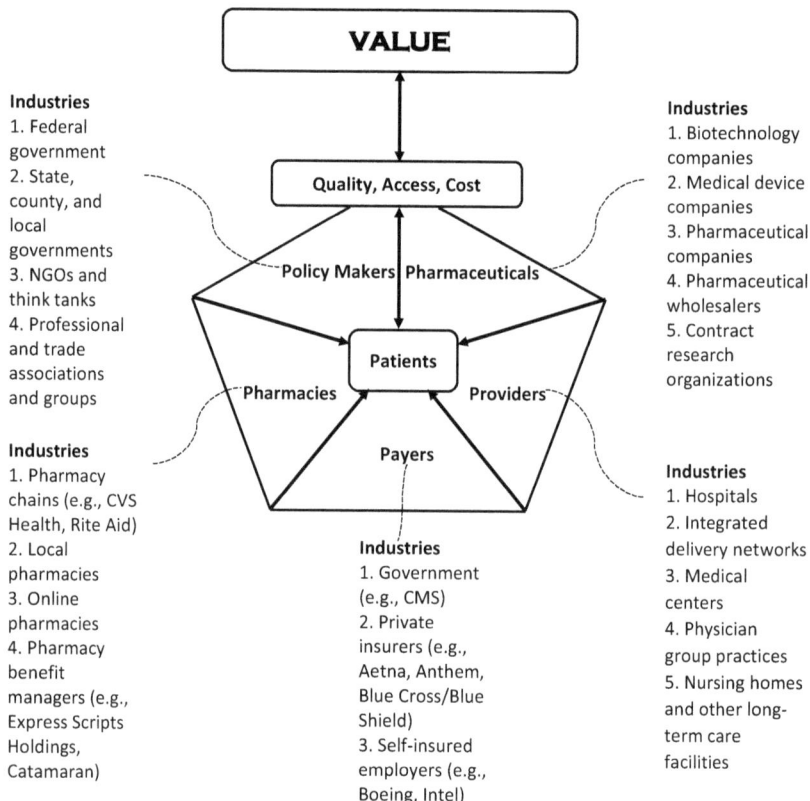

Figure 1.3 The 6 Ps pentagonal framework for health care
Source: Gillespie and Privitera (2018)

---

[10] Gillespie and Privitera, *Patient-Centric Analytics*.

- Providers
- Pharmacies
- Pharmaceuticals
- Payers

Using the 6 Ps framework, patients are at the center of the model. In terms of the *flow* of health care, this framework follows the patients, who elect the policy makers, who then adopt the policies/guidelines for providers, pharmacies, and pharmaceuticals, with those entities getting reimbursed by the payers at the end of the process. In this way, the full health care lifecycle is represented in the 6 Ps framework. Because each *P* plays a vital role in the health care ecosystem, it is critical to align their interests if health care policy is to succeed.

Patients

Patients are at the heart of health care. Patient perspectives are increasingly important in shaping the decision-making processes for their care and health care policy. This shift toward patient-centered care, also called shared decision-making,[11] affirms that patients have valuable insights into their own health. This shift is reflected in programs such as the Ask Me 3 program, which aims to empower patients to take a more active role in their health care and enhance communication among patients, families, and health care professionals.[12]

Patients play a substantive role in advancing health care policy as well. For example, patient advocacy groups play a crucial role in influencing health care policy decisions. These organizations represent the collective voice of patients, often advocating for improved access to care, research funding, and policy changes that benefit specific patient populations.[13] Patient perspectives and feedback serve as a valuable tool for health care providers and policy makers to enhance the quality of patient care, address service gaps, and improve overall patient satisfaction.[14] While the importance of patient involvement in health care policy is widely recognized, there are key challenges to implementing truly patient-centric approaches. These include: ensuring diverse representation of patient voices, managing potential conflicts of interest, balancing patient preferences with evidence-based practices, and standardizing methods for collecting and integrating patient feedback into policy decisions.

---

[11] Montori et al., "Shared Decision-Making."
[12] Institute for Health Care Improvement, "Patient Safety Essentials Toolkit."
[13] Abersone, "Patient Advocacy."   [14] Berger, Saut, and Berssaneti, "Using Patient Feedback."

As health care systems continue to evolve, the role of patients in shaping policy is likely to expand further. Suitably, by fostering a collaborative approach between patients and the other players in the system (i.e., the other 5 *P*s), health care systems can work toward achieving patient-centered care that reflects the needs and values of the populations they serve.

Policy Makers

Policy makers are institutions or groups with the authority to directly impact governmental policies affecting the health care system's operations. They have a wide range of responsibilities that significantly impact the health care landscape and play a vital role in shaping, implementing, and evaluating health care policy.[15] The role of policy makers in health care policy includes:

- Policy development in terms of *setting the agenda* (based on public needs, political feasibility, and evidence from health data), *legislation and regulation* (by drafting, proposing, and enacting laws and regulations that govern health care), and *stakeholder engagement* (by consulting with various stakeholders in health care to gather input and build consensus on health policies).
- Policy implementation in terms of *resource allocation* (including funding for health programs, infrastructure, and research to ensure that financial and human resources are effectively distributed to implement health policies), *program development* (to operationalize health policies by creating specific initiatives such as public health campaigns, insurance programs, and health services), and *regulatory oversight* (by overseeing the enforcement of health regulations and standards, ensuring that health care providers and organizations comply with laws designed to protect patient safety and to promote quality care).
- Policy evaluation in terms of *monitoring and evaluations* (to establish systems to monitor and evaluate the effectiveness of health policies and programs), and *feedback and adjustment* (to ensure that health policies remain relevant and effective over time by evaluating results and stakeholder feedback to make necessary adjustments to policies and programs).

Other ways in which policy makers impact health policy are through advocacy and communication, collaboration and coordination across

---

[15] Rovner, "Congress and the Executive Branch."

different levels of government (local, state, and federal), considering ethical and legal issues, and crisis management (such as during a pandemic). Ultimately, a primary function of health policy makers is to create and implement laws and regulations that govern a health care system.[16] By enacting legislation and establishing regulatory guidelines, policy makers can directly influence how health care is delivered and accessed by a population. In this way, the ability for the United States to pass laws capable of establishing a uniform, universal health care system will require the action and leadership of policy makers.

Providers

Health Care providers play a vital role in health care policy. They are at the point-of-service in the health care system by interacting with patients, both directly (e.g., treating an illness) and indirectly (e.g., making health information accessible to patients via flyers and pamphlets). The role of providers in health care policy includes:

- Policy development in terms of providing *expert opinion* (both clinical expertise and firsthand experience), *research and evidence-based insights* (providers help ensure that policies are based on the best available scientific evidence), and *leadership* (including providers in health policy organizations, government agencies, and think tanks).
- Policy implementation in terms of *establishing guidelines* (clinical guidelines and protocols that align with health policies help standardize care and ensure consistency in practice), *education and training* (providers educate and train other health professionals on new policies and best practices), and *providing direct care* (providers implement health policies directly in their daily practice).
- Policy evaluation in terms of *monitoring and feedback* (providers monitor the impact of health policies on patient outcomes and provide valuable feedback on what is working and what needs adjustment), and *quality improvement* (using data and feedback to refine policies and practices to ensure that policies achieve their intended goals).

Other ways in which providers impact health policy are through advocacy (at the patient and professional level), collaboration and communication (in interdisciplinary teams and public health campaigns and initiatives, which help to translate policy into community action), and

---

[16] World Health Organization, "Consensus Statement."

by ensuring adherence to ethical and legal principles, regulations, and standards. Health Care providers are essential to the health policy process. Their involvement applies evidence-based approaches to ensure that policies are not only theoretically sound but are also practically feasible and effective in optimizing health outcomes.

Pharmacies

Pharmacies play a vital role in health care policy through various functions, including medication management, patient care, public health initiatives, and policy advocacy. They dispense and sell medications, prescriptions, and health devices (e.g., syringes, needles), making them more accessible to patients. The role of pharmacies in health care policy includes:

- Patient care in terms of providing *pharmaceutical care* (including counseling on medication use, side effects, and adherence, supporting policies aimed at improving patient education and self-management), *chronic disease management* (assisting in managing chronic diseases like diabetes, hypertension, and asthma, aligning with health policies that emphasize disease prevention and management), and *vaccinations* (supporting public health initiatives and policies aimed at increasing vaccination rates).
- Medication management in terms of *dispensing medications* (pivotal in implementing policies related to drug distribution by adhering to regulatory standards and ensuring patient safety), offering *Medication Therapy Management (MTM)* (to identify, prevent, and resolve medication-related problems, which contributes to policy goals of safe and effective medication use), and *formulary management* (developing and managing drug formularies, or lists, ensures that patients have access to essential medications as dictated by health care policies).
- Implementation and compliance in terms of *regulatory compliance* (with health policies and regulations, including controlled-substance laws, medication safety standards, and reporting requirements), and *quality assurance* (through the implementation of programs that are aligned with health policies aimed at ensuring high-quality standards of care and medication safety).

Other ways in which pharmacies impact health policy are through public health initiatives (health screenings, preventive services, and health promotion and education), advocacy (at a professional, regulatory, and health care reform level), data collection and reporting (such as through pharmacovigilance programs that contribute to policy development and evaluation by providing insights into medication usage patterns, patient outcomes, and public health trends), collaboration (with health care providers and through referral systems that support policies that promote comprehensive and continuous care), and crisis management (ensuring continuity of medication supply and providing emergency health services during crises). Pharmacies are essential players in the health care policy landscape. Their role ensures that health policies are effectively translated into practice, improving patient outcomes, and contributing to the overall functionality of the health care system.

Pharmaceuticals

Pharmaceutical companies play a significant and multifaceted role in health care policy. Their influence spans drug development, devices, regulation, pricing, accessibility, innovation, and public health. The role of pharmaceuticals in health care policy includes:

- Drug development and implementation in terms of *research and development (R&D)* (driving innovation to discover, develop, and bring new drugs and devices to market), *clinical trials* (to test the efficacy and safety of new drugs, which are essential for regulatory approval and to inform health care policies regarding new treatments and treatment protocols), and through *academic and research partnerships* (aligning with policies that promote scientific research and innovation).
- Pricing and reimbursement in terms of *drug pricing strategies* (drug prices are based on various factors, including R&D costs, market competition, and therapeutic value, which impact patient access to medications and health care costs), *negotiations with payers* (to secure reimbursement for their products, which can impact the inclusion of drugs in formularies and patient access), and through *value-based pricing* (in which drug prices are linked to the clinical outcomes they deliver, which aligns with policies aimed at improving the cost-effectiveness of health care).
- Accessibility and distribution in terms of *global health initiatives* (such as programs like tiered pricing, donations, and public–private partnerships to support global health policies aimed at improving access to essential medicines in underdeveloped countries), and *supply chain management* (to ensure the timely availability of medications, supporting policies aimed at ensuring a reliable supply of essential drugs).

Other ways in which pharmaceuticals impact health policy are through advocacy (by actively lobbying and collaborating with governmental and nongovernmental organizations to support health policies and initiatives that promote public health and access to medications), regulation (to comply with stringent regulatory requirements set by national and global regulatory bodies), public health and education (such as through disease awareness campaigns and patient support programs), ethical considerations (to adhere to ethical standards in research and clinical trials), corporate social responsibility (such as health care outreach, environmental sustainability efforts, and community support, aligning with broader health policy goals), and crisis preparedness (in developing and distributing vaccines and treatments, and supporting emergency health policies and response strategies). Pharmaceutical companies are at the front lines of innovation, making them a key part of the health care landscape. Their role is crucial in translating health policies into practical outcomes that improve patient care, enhance public health, and foster medical advancements.

Payers

Payers play a central role in shaping health care policy, influencing access, affordability, quality of care, and overall health system efficiency. They provide insurance and payment to offset health care expenses for patients, thereby playing a substantive role in the *costs* of health care. The role of payers in health care policy includes:

- Policy development in terms of *benefit design* (with benefit packages that determine the scope of coverage that affects patient access to care and impacts health policies aimed at promoting comprehensive coverage), *payment models* (various payment models, such as fee-for-service, capitation, and value-based payment, influence provider behavior and support policies aimed at improving quality of care and cost-effectiveness), and through *risk management* (by setting premiums and reserves to align with regulatory requirements and actuarial standards that ensure financial stability and compliance with health insurance policies).
- Implementation of health policies in terms of *coverage decisions* (by deciding which treatments, medications, and services are covered, directly influencing patient access to care and potential out-of-pocket costs for essential health coverage), *provider networks* (network management supports policies promoting patient choice and access to high-quality

providers), and through *claims processing* (ensures timely reimbursement for providers and financial protection for patients to align with policies for administrative simplification and efficiency).
- Financial protection and access to care in terms of *premium subsidies and assistance programs* (to make coverage more affordable for low-income individuals and families, aligning with policies aimed at expanding access to insurance), and *catastrophic coverage* (to protect patients from financial ruin due to major health events, aligning with policies designed to provide financial protection and reduce medical bankruptcy).

Other ways in which payers impact health policy are through advocacy (to influence health care legislation and regulation related to insurance markets, health benefits, and payment reforms), compliance (to ensure that their operations align with legal standards), quality improvement (through programs incentivizing providers to meet performance benchmarks and improve patient outcomes), care coordination (to manage patient care across multiple providers and settings to reduce fragmentation and support policies promoting integrated and patient-centered care), reporting and analytics (through health data analysis and reporting to assess the effectiveness of interventions, and provide data to regulatory bodies and stakeholders, supporting policies aimed at accountability and informed decision-making), and preventative care and health promotion (by covering preventive services and implementing health promotion initiatives to encourage healthy behaviors and lifestyle choices that align with policies promoting population health and wellness). Payers are integral to the health care policy ecosystem. By collaborating with providers, policy makers, and other stakeholders, insurers can contribute to a more effective and equitable health care environment.

1.5 Across the Pond: How Are Health and Diversity Related?

In a single hour at a clinic, a health care provider might encounter an older construction worker suffering from back pain, a young family concerned about how they will cover their medical expenses, a teenager managing mental health issues, and a patient who is transgender seeking a routine checkup. Even without mentioning race, we can see that health care is diverse in its very nature. With the United States also becoming more racially and ethnically diverse over the last decade,[17] it's increasingly clear that national health care policy must be inclusive of the diversity of those it serves.

---

[17] Jones et al., "Race and Ethnicity Measures."

Diversity, which encompasses the unique characteristics and perspectives of individuals in a population, is largely seen as a barrier to health care.[18] To take a closer look at *how* diversity can be a barrier, let's consider the diversity by race/ethnicity of the top thirty-five healthiest nations in the world, listed in Table 1.3.

Health rankings are measured using the **Bloomberg Global Health Index**,[19] which is a holistic measure of national health that includes many factors such as health risks (e.g., obesity), average life expectancy, and living conditions (e.g., water quality). It is scored as a value between 0 and 100, with larger values indicating better health. The diversity of a nation is measured using the **Fractionalization Index**,[20] which is a measure of the likelihood that two people selected at random in a given population will be from two different groups. It is scored as a value between 0 and 100, with larger values indicating greater diversity. Table 1.2 shows the Fractionalization Index score for two different ethnic groups, by nation.

Referring to Table 1.3, it is striking how health and diversity rankings differ. Among the top ten healthiest nations, only three are inside the top 100 for racial diversity. Among the top thirty-five healthiest nations, less than half (fourteen nations) are inside the top 100 for racial diversity. If we compute a Spearman correlation for the rankings of the top thirty-five healthiest countries, we find a negative correlation ($r = -0.33$) with greater racial diversity being related to lower health rankings. In total, 11 percent of the variability in health rankings can be explained by the racial diversity of a given nation. The takeaway: Racial diversity is a key barrier to achieving better national health outcomes.

Let us appeal to the common adage: *correlation is not causation*. When considering diversity, it is important, at a policy level, to consider what factors are related to being more diverse as a nation, particularly in terms of how policy can positively affect health. For example, diversity at an individual level reflects a person's distinct background, beliefs, values, and health care needs that are shaped by their cultural heritage. This diversity of individuals necessitates a personalized approach rather than a standardized care model to avoid isolating patients.[21] Key cultural factors to consider for shaping health policy include:

---

[18] Centers for Disease Control and Prevention (CDC), "Ambulatory Care Use."
[19] World Population Review, "Healthiest Countries 2024."
[20] World Population Review, "Most Racially Diverse Countries."
[21] Younas et al., "Sociocultural and Patient-Healthcare."

Table 1.3 *The score and ranking for health and ethnic diversity of a nation*

Country	Bloomberg Global Health Index	Rank	Fractionalization Index (HIEF 2013)	Rank
Spain	92.75	1	0.67	41
Italy	91.59	2	0.11	142
Iceland	91.44	3	0.00	185
Japan	91.38	4	1.90	154
Switzerland	90.93	5	36.70	92
Sweden	90.24	6	21.90	120
Australia	89.75	7	27.60	107
Singapore	89.29	8	39.50	86
Norway	89.09	9	15.10	136
Israel	88.15	10	37.60	87
Luxembourg	87.39	11	0.00	165
France	86.94	12	0.00	183
Austria	86.30	13	27.60	107
Finland	85.89	14	13.80	138
Netherlands	85.86	15	35.40	95
Cameroon	85.70	16	0.00	155
South Korea	85.41	17	9.50	145
United Kingdom	84.28	18	39.90	82
Ireland	84.06	19	17.40	130
Cyprus	83.58	20	34.70	97
Portugal	83.10	21	22.00	119
Germany	83.06	22	18.90	126
Slovenia	82.72	23	25.80	111
Denmark	82.69	24	17.70	128
Greece	82.29	25	16.70	132
Malta	81.70	26	0.00	190
Belgium	80.46	27	59.20	53
Czech Republic	77.59	28	26.20	109
Cuba	74.66	29	51.70	70
Croatia	73.36	30	17.10	131
Estonia	73.32	31	45.80	75
Chile	73.21	32	43.90	79
Costa Rica	73.21	33	39.80	83
United States	73.02	34	52.70	67
Bahrain	72.31	35	58.20	57

- Family and community, which play a crucial role in shaping an individual's beliefs and perceptions, especially in certain cultures. In some communities, the interests of the family take precedence over those of the individual, influencing the health care decision-making process.

- Religious beliefs can pose barriers to certain treatments or involve dietary restrictions, requiring accommodation in health care plans.
- Perspectives on death and end-of-life care vary across cultures, necessitating culturally sensitive approaches.
- Gender roles and dynamics within relationships can impact health care decisions and willingness to seek treatment.
- Cultural beliefs about health, pain tolerance, and the efficacy of different treatments can influence patient expectations and adherence to treatment plans.
- Genetic and physiological factors may result in varying responses to medication among different cultural groups, impacting treatment outcomes. This feature of culture is part of the exciting growth of personalized medicine.

Health Care systems and policies that are capable of addressing diversity differ across countries, which influences the role of patients. Some nations have decentralized or collaborative approaches to health care planning, involving various stakeholders, while others have more centralized systems. Funding mechanisms for health care can also vary, including general taxation, national health insurance, private insurance, out-of-pocket payments, and charitable donations. The presence or absence of universal health care coverage can likewise impact access and equity for patients. All of these systems and policies impact a nation's ability to close health disparity gaps and reduce barriers to care.

1.6 Moving toward a Healthy Society

The scope of this book is focused on what we refer to as the *axes of the US health care debate*: government and equity. We address government in terms of its involvement in health care, with the perspective that data from the healthiest countries in the world affirms the need for government involvement in health care to ensure access for all. We address equity by asking, "Is the health care debate in the US too focused on insurance for all?" While access to health care is essential, the social determinants of health account for about 80 percent of the variability in quality-of-life and length-of-life measures (as introduced at the beginning of this chapter and illustrated in Figure 1.1). For this reason, to achieve health equity, we must go further than simply guaranteeing health insurance for everyone by also addressing the social determinants *in health care policy*. Suitably, as we dive deeper into the features of health care and health care policy, we present, in this book, a focused, data-driven discussion for these two critical, yet related, policy constraints in the US health care debate.

Chapter Summary

This introductory chapter emphasizes the importance of viewing health care policy as beyond merely providing access to doctors. While quality health care is vital, social determinants – such as economic stability, education, and neighborhood environments – play a more substantial role in determining health outcomes. These external factors account for approximately 80 percent of life quality and longevity, underscoring the need for health care policies to address broader societal inequities. Equity, equality, and justice are explored as approaches to reducing health disparities. While equality ensures uniform resource distribution and equity customizes support to individual needs, justice aims to eliminate systemic barriers, offering sustainable solutions. Examples like equitable COVID-19 vaccine distribution underscore the importance of justice-driven policies in reducing health disparities and fostering long-term population health equity.

The chapter also elucidates the fragmented US health care system, which incorporates elements of four global models: Beveridge, Bismarck, National Health Insurance, and out-of-pocket. This fragmentation creates inefficiencies and inequities in access, quality, and costs, measured through tools like the Donabedian model and the HAQ Index. The 6 Ps framework – patients, policy makers, providers, pharmacies, pharmaceuticals, and payers – illustrates the complex interplay of stakeholders in the health care system. To improve US health care, it is important to align interests across the 6 Ps to ensure that all people have *access* to *quality* care that they can afford (*costs*).

CHAPTER 2

Paying the Most, Getting the Least

Insights

- Americans pay the most and get the least of any nation in the world for health care.
- Many Americans unnecessarily experience shorter, sicker lives.
- The United States does not have a health spending problem. It has a health value problem.
- The United States excels at care processes and preventative care.
- The cost per unit is a bigger problem than total utilization in the US health care system.

A principal obligation of a government is to safeguard the health and welfare of its citizens. To this end, every health system aims to provide accessible, low-cost, quality care. In this regard, how is the US health care system performing? Overall, as we will discuss, the performance is decidedly mixed. Reform is widely acknowledged as being needed regarding access to primary care, affordability, insurance coverage, and system efficiency. The United States can learn valuable lessons from others about how to improve our health care delivery and outcomes.

Each country has a unique health care system that has evolved over decades and perhaps even centuries, impacted by a myriad of cultural, economic, political, social, and technological changes. Thus, one always has to be circumspect in comparative international analysis. Still, by most independent measures, with regard to its health care system, the United States is an outlier, but not in a good way. The US public health system is fractured. The expression that the United States has a "sickcare" system rather than a health care system has been used to a sufficient degree as to be trite, but it unfortunately remains true. Over time, the United States will need to move closer in performance to peer nations to remain competitive economically as Americans are currently not getting the best value for their health care dollar.

2.1 Comparative Analysis of the US Health Care System

Since health care is so complex, macro assessment of overall system performance can be difficult. There are at least three basic ways of working toward this. First, one method is to compare the current performance of the US health care system against the past performance of the US health care system (i.e., trendline analysis). This has the advantage of holding certain unique features of the United States constant (e.g., constitutional democracy with a federated governmental structure). The challenge is that many variables naturally change over time (e.g., growth in the internet and more phone usage, changes to ethnic/racial demographics, advances in medical technologies, the advent of COVID-19). A second method is to measure the current actual performance of the US health care system against a theoretical maximum possibility (i.e., constrained optimization modeling, which is typically done by computer simulations). How should the system work and what would it look like if effectiveness and efficiency were optimized? This kind of modeling can yield valuable predictive and prescriptive analysis, and with the growth of AI, deep learning, and machine learning, the capabilities in this regard are continually growing. The challenge is that care and medicine are often so complex, uncertain, emotional, visceral, and human as to be resistant to tidy computer modeling. A third method is to measure the performance of the US health care system against the performance of peer countries (i.e., benchmarking analysis). This has the significant advantage of comparing identical periods of time, which serves to hold a variety of key factors (e.g., a global pandemic or a global recession) relatively constant. The challenge is the sheer variety of differences between countries. However, most health care researchers have adopted this third approach, as do we. It provides the most rigorous assessment and the most relevant points of comparison.

Almost like human DNA, every nation has a truly individualized health care system reflecting its own complicated cultural, economic, legal, political, social, and technological circumstances, yet comparison can still be quite useful for policymaking. The Organisation for Economic Co-operation and Development's (OECD) 2024 health statistics report provides a comprehensive analysis of how the US health care system compares to other countries.[1] The US health care system continues to underperform even while spending at high rates, ranking last in overall performance when compared to nine other wealthy countries: Australia, Canada, France, Germany, the Netherlands, New Zealand, Sweden, Switzerland, and the United Kingdom.[2] The key criteria

---

[1] OECD, "OECD Health Statistics." [2] Blumenthal et al., "Mirror, Mirror 2024."

were access to care, administrative efficiency, care processes, equity in care, and outcomes. The top performers globally include Australia, the Netherlands, and the United Kingdom. Similarly, the Netherlands, the UK, and Germany ranked first, second, and third, respectively, in a Commonwealth Fund study, with the United States lagging behind.[3]

Not surprisingly, wealthier countries generally tend to spend more on average for everything (e.g., art, entertainment, health care, infrastructure, transportation) than poorer countries. Thus, the fact that the United States, which is the richest country in the world, spends more on health care than any other nation is not particularly shocking. The disconcerting – and surprising – element is the lack of value gained for the dollars spent. The United States spends on health care like the wealthy country that it is but gets outcomes like a poor country that it is not. The United States spends over $13,000 per person on health care, which is the highest cost per capita compared to similar countries. For example, Switzerland is the second highest-spending country per capita, but only equals just over $9,000, so the United States is spending about $4,000 per person more than any other country in the world.[4] The US outcomes are worse in areas like infant mortality, life expectancy, and unmanaged diabetes.

Figure 2.1 nicely captures how life expectancy combined with expenditure yields poor value for the United States.

The United States Has the Lowest Life Expectancy Among Large, Wealthy Countries While Far Outspending Them on Health Care

Life expectancy (2021) and per capita health care spending (2021 or nearest year)

Country	Life expectancy	Health spending, per capita
United States	76.1	$12,318
United Kingdom	80.8	$5,387
Germany	80.9	$7,383
Austria	81.3	$6,693
Netherlands	81.5	$6,190
Belgium	81.9	$5,274
Comparable Country Average	82.4	$6,003
France	82.5	$5,468
Sweden	83.2	$6,262
Australia	83.4	$5,627
Switzerland	84.0	$7,179
Japan	84.5	$4,666

Figure 2.1 Life expectancy and expenditure
Source: Kaiser Family Foundation

[3] Blumenthal et al., "Mirror, Mirror 2024." [4] OECD, "OECD Health Statistics."

The US health care system's pattern of spending the most but getting the least is not economically, fiscally, or medically sustainable.

2.2 US Spending on Health Care: Price per Unit versus Total Utilization

The United States has long been a big, diverse country, and many of its core democratic and economic principles have remained relatively constant, yet it was only toward the end of the twentieth century that the United States became an outlier on health care expenditures. Thus, with regard to the health care system, there is no reason to believe that the current state of spending the most and getting the least is inherently endemic to the United States. In theory at least, the system can be changed to bring the US health care a return on investment or ROI (i.e., [access + quality]/cost) in line with peer nations.

In 1970, about 7 percent of the US gross domestic product (GDP) went toward health care costs, which is somewhat higher than but not radically different from the 5 percent average that similarly wealthy countries spent. In the intervening five decades, and especially beginning in the 1980s, that difference grew substantially, with the United States spending on health care ballooning to over 18 percent of GDP while other countries remained relatively constant.[5] Over the next decade, US health spending is projected to increase an average of 5.4 percent per year, outpacing annual projected GDP growth, and by 2031, health care spending is expected to consume 19.6 percent of GDP.[6]

At its simplest, total health spending is driven by a function of utilization multiplied by price per unit. Holding all else constant, spending rises when there is an increase in the number of services used and/or an increase in the cost charged per service. Ironically, the utilization rates in the United States are relatively similar to other advanced, industrialized wealthy nations.[7] Thus, despite frequent media reports, as well as some structural dynamics (e.g., insurance plans with low or no **copays** and **deductibles**), overuse is not the principal problem in the US health care system. To be sure, as we note elsewhere, there are often a few heavy users (e.g., patients with costly comorbidities) who can consume a sizable portion of health care services. However, those individuals are often "balanced out" by

---

[5] Wager and Cox, "International Comparison."
[6] Keehan et al., "National Health Expenditure Projections."
[7] Kamal and Cox, "Healthcare Prices."

people who under-consume services (e.g., avoiding annual physical exams, failing to get preventative procedures, delaying medically recommended surgeries like angioplasties). Also, patients in the United States tend to have shorter hospital stays, which produces substantial net cost savings. The real "villain" in the United States is the price per service rendered, rather than utilization. For example, administrative costs in the United States exceed $1,000 per person, which is a whopping five times the average of other wealthy nations. The United States also spends significantly more on long-term care.

Thus, the United States does not really have a health care cost or a health care spending problem per se. In the abstract, there is nothing necessarily disadvantageous to public health, governmental fiscal stability, or societal economic welfare by there being a high per capita spending on health care. Instead, at its core, the United States has a value problem. The ratio of access and quality (i.e., the numerator) to costs (i.e., the denominator) is comparatively unfavorable. One way to address this is the common argument for lowering the denominator – do everything possible to drive down costs. However, another way is to increase the numerator – use the money being spent to substantially broaden access and raise quality. In fact, both approaches should be undertaken.

The United States spends about $7,500 per person on inpatient and outpatient care, compared to about $3,900 in peer nations.[8] The overall higher total cost is driven more by this price per unit differential rather than utilization per person. Patients in the United States tend to receive a great intensity of treatment per interaction, including access to and utilization of advanced diagnostic and treatment technologies, which tend to be relatively more expensive. The United States spends about $1,700 per capita annually on prescription drugs (along with over-the-counter drugs and medical equipment) and about $950 on health care administration.[9] Drivers of health costs include discrimination, drug abuse, gun violence, homelessness, hunger, and poverty. For example, last year, the United States experienced more than 100,000 drug overdose deaths[10] and over 43,000 gun-related fatalities.[11] It is commonly assumed that the United States can solve its health care value issue solely by some combination of reducing the price of prescription drugs and restraining administrative costs. These are certainly laudable goals, but together, they

---

[8] Wager and Cox, "International Comparison." [9] Wager and Cox, "International Comparison."
[10] National Center for Health Statistics, *U.S. Overdose Deaths Decrease*.
[11] Washburn, "Gun Violence."

only constitute a subset of total costs. The primary solutions have to focus on the direct costs of inpatient and outpatient care, while still working to reduce the costs of prescriptions and administration.

2.3 Accessibility and Affordability

As a first step, we need a system that is accessible and affordable. The highest-quality health care is not broadly meaningful if only a few can both access and afford it. Accessibility and affordability are distinct but often are closely interrelated. Access to health care is the ultimate Achilles' heel for the US system. There are over 25 million completely uninsured Americans and tens of millions more who have high out-of-pocket costs that make utilization financially unattractive.[12] In sharp contrast, countries such as Germany and the Netherlands are characterized by affordable care and universal coverage.

There is no other country in the world where patients, families, and caregivers are expected to pay as much out of pocket for their core health care. Patients often need medications they cannot afford. Even "fully" insured Americans struggle financially with health care costs. Given that nearly 25 percent of Americans report skipping medication but only 9.2 percent of the US population is uninsured, this vividly tells us that having at least some form of insurance is not the complete answer. The missing element here is that insurance needs to make it so that actually consuming the health care is (i) affordable and (ii) convenient. In contrast, in Austria, Czechia, Germany, and the Netherlands, less than 0.5 percent of the population reports unmet needs for medical care.[13]

The profound complexity of the US insurance system imposes additional financial and nonfinancial burdens on both patients and providers, generating administrative inefficiencies unmatched in peer nations. Other countries do a better job at simplifying the complexity of health insurance, investing in accessible primary care, and providing more public health-oriented education and training for providers. The US health care system is particularly – perhaps even peculiarly – complex, with a byzantine mix of public and private payers offering thousands of health plans with unique provider networks, coverage limitations, and cost-sharing requirements.

As part of this complexity, health care providers experience challenges with both insurance approvals and service billing, with patients' care often

---

[12] Hale et al., "Health Insurance Coverage Projections."
[13] Eurostat, "Unmet Healthcare Needs Statistics."

delayed or their claims denied. Physicians and their staff often consume valuable time in back-and-forth exchanges with insurance companies regarding care authorization, especially when there is a denial. Many countries have taken steps to greatly simplify their health insurance, billing, and payment systems. This can be done through governmental legislation/regulation or industry codification/standardization.

In thinking about access, in addition to affordability, the United States could also use a more robust primary care system. For example, in most countries, a **primary care physician (PCP)** is typically available after normal business hours. In the United States, that is typically not the case. Instead, most after-hour care is managed by an emergency room or urgent care provider, with the PCP usually brought into the process part way through. Emergency room care tends to be expensive, decontextualized, and less relationship oriented. The resulting bill process is often more convoluted than if care has been managed through one's primary doctor. Aggravating the access issues, the United States also has a physician shortage with just 2.7 practicing physicians per 1,000 people, compared to an average of 3.9 in comparable countries.[14] Moreover, the gap is wider for PCPs, who compose only 12 percent of physicians in the United States.

2.4 Equity and Disparities

Health disparities (also known as health inequities) are differences in health diagnoses, processes, and outcomes between different subpopulations. By 2050, people of color are projected to account for over half (52 percent) of the US population, with the largest increases occurring with people who identify as Asian or Hispanic,[15] so this is going to become an increasingly important dynamic. The United States generally scores relatively poorly on health equity, with substantial access disparities related to race and ethnicity, including many anecdotal and objective reports of discrimination. The problem in the United States was shown vividly during the COVID-19 crisis and is summarized by this graph in Figure 2.2.

In the Commonwealth Fund report, the United States performed poorly on health inequities related to race and ethnicity, and it was also characterized by the highest income-related difference in access.[16] Thus, health equity has a profound socioeconomic dimension; refer to Figure 2.3.

---

[14] Medford-Davis et al., "Physician Shortage."
[15] United States Census Bureau, *2023 National Population Projections.*
[16] Blumenthal et al., "Mirror, Mirror 2024."

2.4 Equity and Disparities

During the pandemic, premature deaths among people of color resulted in more years of life lost than among White people

Average years of life lost per premature excess death under the age of seventy-five during the COVID-19 pandemic, by race/ethnicity, March 28, 2020 to December 31, 2022

AIAN	22.0
Hispanic	21.0
NHOPI	18.8
Black	18.3
All groups	15.6
Asian	14.0
White	12.5

Figure 2.2 People of color more likely to die
Source: Kaiser Family Foundation

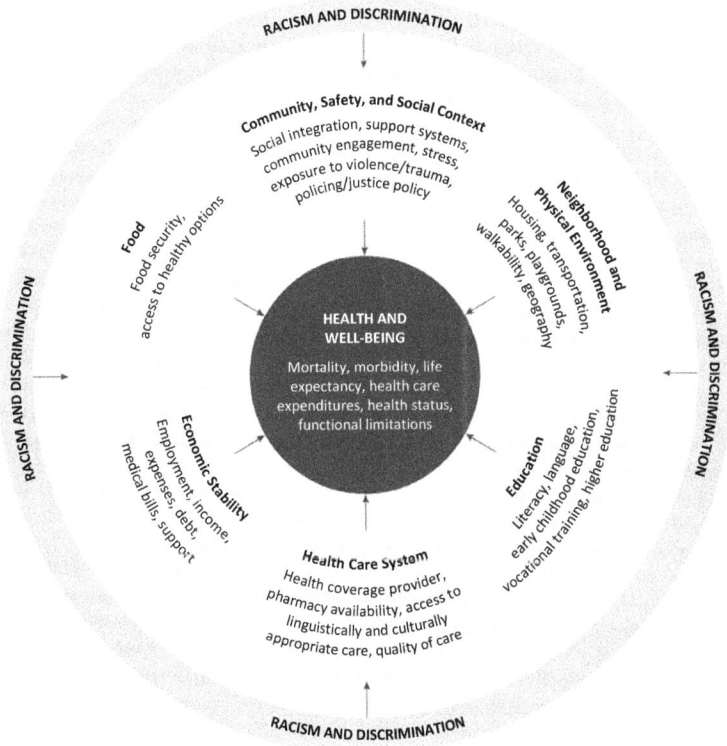

Figure 2.3 Health disparities
Source: Kaiser Family Foundation

Other sources of disparities are citizenship status and gender/sexual identity and orientation. Because of the frequent multiplicity of people's identities, many patients experience disparities across more than one dimension.

Not all differences are caused by disparities. For example, the elderly (post seventy years old) typically have more falls than a middle-aged adult (forty to sixty years old) and are slower to recover. These different outcomes are not caused by the identity or relative social standing of these elderly; they are typically simply a function of the body naturally growing more fragile as humans age. At the same time, older patients can fall victim to ageism, which is a type of disparity. Disparities can occur along a number of lines: age, disability, ethnicity, gender, geography, race, sexual orientation, socioeconomic status, or veteran status. Addressing health disparities is integral to improvements in the overall society. Not only is it the right thing to do from a fairness perspective, but it is also good medicine, good public health, and good public policy.

Mental health care is another important dimension of disparities. Over 20 percent of US adults experienced a mental illness annually, and almost 5 percent of all adult Americans reported serious thoughts of suicide.[17] Yet, approximately 5.5 million adults with mental illness are uninsured, causing many to forego badly needed treatment.[18] In fact, many experts argue that the United States is experiencing mental health crises that have only worsened in the aftermath of COVID-19. There remains a need to expand Medicaid coverage for mental health services, while reducing discrimination and stigma.

In the past couple of decades, there has been an increased focus on the social determinants of health (SDOH) such as crime and violence, food insecurity, housing insecurity, and poor nutrition. As part of this, we know it is essential to expand social safety nets to catch those uninsured and underinsured "**frequent flyers**" who often drive a disproportionate share of health care costs, but to at least some extent, SDOH dynamics apply to almost everyone. We return to this topic in the next chapter.

2.5 Not All Gloom and Doom: Areas Where the United States Excels

The United States does rank fairly high in care process. This is a strength to build upon. The elements of care process include prevention, safety, coordination, patient engagement, and sensitivity to patient preferences.

---

[17] Mental Health America, "Statistics about Mental Health."
[18] Mental Health America, "Statistics about Mental Health."

2.5 Not All Gloom and Doom: Where the US Excels

The United States performs relatively well on this index. And why does it rank so highly? Four likely reasons. First, it has a strong emphasis on patient safety and many preventative procedures (e.g., flu vaccinations, mammograms, colonoscopies). Second, the patient experience is often tracked and monitored via surveys, and as importantly, there are concrete metrics attached to the results. Third, perhaps via some combination of the fear of government oversight, insurance company denials/nonpayment, and patient lawsuits, US providers are generally compelled/motivated to be attentive to process. Fourth, the shift from volume-based to value-based care, while still uneven in its impact, has generally caused payers to more strongly emphasize incentive-based performance, which has positively altered provider behavior.

Over the past fifteen years, the United States has experienced a reduction in adverse events (e.g., infections) for a variety of hospital-required stays (e.g., major surgeries).[19] This reflects a concerted effort by government, nongovernmental organizations, and the private sector to emphasize patient safety. One positive factor is that the United States spends more on preventative care than other countries with a similar GDP. This includes disease detection, education, emergency preparedness, mass immunizations, and preventive health programs. Also positive from a fiscal perspective, the United States spends less per capita on long-term care compared to most other peer nations. This includes health and social services offered by long-term care institutions (e.g., nursing homes, home-based settings, and community-based settings).

While US hospital stays are relatively low, which is generally a positive factor, that comes at the cost of more extensive and intensive outpatient care. Second, one finds evidence from comparative studies of well-defined procedures and patient populations that the United States provides more services in settings that are not as consistently tracked in the OECD data across countries, such as post-acute care or specialty outpatient care, especially for high-need patients. In fact, the relatively low US lengths of stay are consistent with a greater push to post-acute care via a variety of often quite intensive ambulatory settings. So, for US society overall, it is a bit of pay me now (through hospital care) or pay me later (through ambulatory care). The net is likely lower because hospitals are relatively expensive, but overall cost savings within the care episode are not as significant as one would think.

---

[19] Eldridge et al., "Adverse Event Rates."

The United States is widely acknowledged as a global leader in health care technology. Relatively recent technologies such as artificial intelligence, electronic health records, and telemedicine are increasingly being developed, yet the ultimate impact of these tools is still unknown. For example, many physicians and patients complain that electronic medical record input requirements during the session actively impair the treatment relationship.[20] Unfortunately, advanced technology can often be a cost driver rather than a generator of savings. US providers conduct about 45 percent more magnetic resonance imaging exams and 62 percent more computed tomography scans compared to the OECD average.[21] The US rate of coronary artery bypass graft surgery was also over 50 percent higher for patients with acute myocardial infarction relative to other nations.[22] We need an active vision for how technology can reduce rather than neutrally or even negatively impact health expenditures.

2.6 Across the Pond: Health Care Insurance Uncovered, Nonuniversal

Despite significant measures such as the Medicare (for adults aged sixty-five and older) and Medicaid (for low-income patients) programs adopted in 1965 and the Affordable Care Act passed in 2010, as well as the popularity of employer-driven coverage, the US system today rests on a largely volunteer foundation, which leaves tens of millions with no or insufficient insurance. Among advanced industrialized countries, the United States is striking for its lack of universal coverage. In other countries, health care is generally accessible and affordable, with relatively low copays, but in the United States, about 7–8 percent of the population is completely uninsured.[23] This is a good news, bad news story. This rate is actually very low by historical US standards as there has been a positive trend line on coverage (positive). However, the United States still lags significantly behind relative to peer nations (negative).

No country relies to the extent the United States does upon a largely unregulated private market to allocate essential health care resources. Almost half of all Americans get their health care via an employer.[24] Due to the sharp increase in private plan deductibles, about 25 percent of the working-age population is essentially underinsured. High

---

[20] Honavar, "Electronic Medical Records." [21] Papanicolas et al., "Healthcare Spending."
[22] Cram et al., "Variation in Revascularisation Use."
[23] U.S. Department of Health and Human Services, *National Uninsured Rate*.
[24] Hale et al., "Health Insurance Coverage Projections."

copays, deductibles, and other cost-sharing/cost-shifting arrangements suppress valid demand for medical treatment. This results in behavior (e.g., skipping medical tests, avoiding treatments, failing to fill prescriptions) that is likely to be counterproductive to effective care and sound health.

It is a common mistake to assume that universal coverage automatically or by definition means one national-level governmental payer. It is usually – and probably correctly – assumed that in the United States a proposal like that would be "dead on arrival" for three reasons. First, it would run into philosophical and political opposition for people who are opponents of "big government" as it would increase public-sector influence, especially at the federal level. Second, many Americans would be forced to give up their **employer-provided insurance** coverage. Third, a public sector–dominant insurance system would squeeze out the economic interests of the current, powerful private-sector insurers.

However, and fortunately, universality can be achieved in a diverse variety of ways, as comparisons to other nations demonstrate. For example, the United Kingdom has a massive health system that is almost exclusively publicly funded and operated, yet other nations such as Switzerland have an extensive compulsory private insurance system. And still other countries include a comprehensive mix of private and public insurance. Moreover, the essence of universal coverage is developing financial mechanisms to eliminate any gaps in insurance coverage for the population. It does not have to radically alter the existing patterns and players that provide the actual health care.

Some comparisons on coverage:

- England: National Health Service provides free public health care, including physician services, hospitalization, and mental health care.
- Germany: Copays capped at 1 percent of gross income for the chronically ill and 2 percent for all others, with all other care covered in full.
- Netherlands: Primary care, maternity care, and childcare fully covered, with all other care covered after payment of a modest annual deductible.

2.7 Disparities in US Health Care: The Need for Positive Change

The troubled US health care system has real consequences: Relative to citizens in peer countries, Americans tend to be sicker, die earlier, and experience more difficulty affording essential care. Many Americans are unnecessarily experiencing shorter, sicker lives because of the health system. The United States is characterized by the most acute illnesses and chronic diseases, and it has the highest per capita rate of avoidable deaths among top wealthy countries. As measured by rates of diabetes, heart disease, hypertension, and obesity, US patients do seem to be sicker than peers around the globe in comparatively wealthy countries. Poor health care leads to premature disability and early deaths.

These severe consequences negatively impact the very old, the very young, and everyone in between. Elderly patients are often sicker than they should be due to a lifetime spent mostly uninsured. The United States has higher maternal and infant death rates than another comparable high-income country. The estimates vary, but it is generally acknowledged that between 8 and 12 million US children live in poverty.[25] For the COVID-19 pandemic, the United States had the highest attributable percentages of excess deaths for people younger than seventy-five years old. While spending about twice as much per person on health costs in comparison to other large, wealthy countries, the United States has seen declining performance on many health outcomes in the wake of the COVID-19 pandemic.[26] The maternal mortality rate for Black mothers is shockingly about three times the rate for White mothers, irrespective of age and socioeconomic groups.[27] And also alarmingly, every racial/ethnic, socioeconomic, and age group in the United States has a higher maternal mortality rate than the average in peer nations.[28] So many mothers are dying during what should be one of the happiest moments of their lives.

In 1980, the 73.7-year life expectancy of the typical American was comparable to the populations of other wealthy nations. However, over the last forty years, the US life expectancy has not kept pace with the continued growth in other countries. Thus, the United States now has a fairly profound death gap: 78.8 years in the United States versus 82.7 years in comparable countries. Given this difference of about four years and taking into account that the annual death rate in the United States is about 3 million,[29] it means that we are needlessly losing over 12 million years of life annually – clearly a suboptimal situation and one that requires the increased governmental attention we will explore in the next chapter.

---

[25] Padilla and Thomson, "Children in Poverty." [26] Wager et al., "U.S. Health System."
[27] Njoku et al., "Black Maternal Mortality." [28] Njoku et al., "Black Maternal Mortality."
[29] Ahmad, Cisewski, and Anderson, "Mortality."

Chapter Summary

In this chapter, we explored the health care needs of the exceptionally diverse nation that is the United States. The United States is characterized by worse levels of disparities and inequalities compared to high-performing health care nations, and this is not solely or even primarily attributable to demographic differences. Moreover, substandard health care often translates into lost employee productivity, and there are additional economic losses attributable to premature deaths. The intercountry comparisons can help inform health care solutions for US policy, and in the next chapter, we focus on several of these, including universal health care coverage.

With health care in the United States, everything is inherently political and partisan. However, as it has been proven by many other advanced industrialized nations, we believe access, affordability, and quality of the US health care system can be improved in commonsense ways that would have broad appeal. The current high costs yet poor outcomes in the US health care system as a whole undermine economic growth and threaten long-term fiscal stability. There are more effective and efficient pathways for patients, providers, payers, pharmaceuticals, pharmacies, and policy makers to pursue together in the effort to effectuate positive change.

CHAPTER 3

Government Drives Access

Insights

- The foundational problem in the US health care system is a misalignment of incentives, including negative and positive externalities.
- There is no universal system or way of achieving universal health care.
- Even insured patients often struggle to access and afford care.
- The private sector is not necessarily more efficient at delivering health care than the public sector.
- One solution to address access challenges is to bring health care directly to patients rather than bringing patients to access health care.

Health, being a matter of both individual responsibility and private insurance, is a foundational principle of the American health care system. This has made movements toward universal health care fraught with acrimony. US health care debates have been characterized by hyper-partisan politics, so efforts to solve problems have become deeply polarizing and often will provoke powerful "special interests" to lobby on one side or another. Health Care lobbying increased 70 percent over the past two decades in the United States,[1] with an estimated 4,500–5,000 health lobbyists per Member of Congress.[2]

Yet, there is overwhelming bipartisan agreement that the current system severely underperforms in many respects. Despite efforts by government agencies, health care organizations, community groups, and corporate groups to improve health care access and overall outcomes in the United States, there remains a profound challenge. The current US health care system is a patchwork hodgepodge that few experts, patients, or policy makers love. Plus, there are significant fraud, abuse, and errors to be found

---

[1] Pifer, "Healthcare Lobbying."   [2] Schpero et al., "Lobbying Expenditures."

in the health care system. We want to employ commonsense, evidence-based solutions to improve health care access.

The Governmental Accounting Office and the Congressional Budget Office both maintain that health care spending is the leading driver of long-term federal government spending and debt accumulation. The increasingly large elderly segment of the population is likely to further stimulate that trend. The American Cancer Society reports that over 55 percent of Americans experience some form of financial hardship attendant to seeking medical care.[3] Health Care costs are the top driver of personal bankruptcy. People in poverty tend to have higher disease burdens. Either poor finances or poor health can trigger a vicious cycle of poverty and poor health outcomes over time.

The debate around health care often trends to the negative, and certainly we can all agree that there is a lot to be concerned with and disappointed by. However, it is also important to employ positive frameworks around health care too. Due to its potential to unlock human capital and pay economic dividends for countries, health should be viewed as an investment rather than as an expense. Could that argument not be made regarding nearly every public expense? Yes. However, health care is one of the best investments we can make because sound health is foundational to individual productivity. So rather than proceeding exclusively from a deficient model framework, there are benefits to assessing health care in terms of what value it adds to the economy and whether it becomes a potential generator of positive return on investment (ROI) for society. Having both a nonpartisan framing and a nonnegative framing would go a long way to improving the quality of debate around health care in the United States.

3.1 Across the Pond: Aligning Incentives in Health Care

The fundamental challenge to be addressed in the US health care system is the misalignment of various incentives, including **negative externalities** (i.e., costs caused by another entity's actions) and **positive externalities** (benefits caused by another entity's actions). The complex marketplace for health care services does not always incentivize institutions to provide better care for more people and it does not always incentivize individuals to take better care for themselves. Health systems, hospitals, and pharmaceutical companies tend to charge what insurance companies will pay

---

[3] Yabroff et al., "Cancer Diagnosis."

rather than what patients can afford. And, for example, there need to be increased incentives for physicians and mental health care professionals to work in underserved locations (e.g., rural areas and the "inner city"). The current system creates inherent market failures with both negative externalities (which cause an over-generation of adverse actions) and positive externalities (which cause an under-generation of advantageous actions) abounding.

Figure 3.1 captures some of this incentive misalignment. We present a few of the many key variables that motivate patients, providers, and

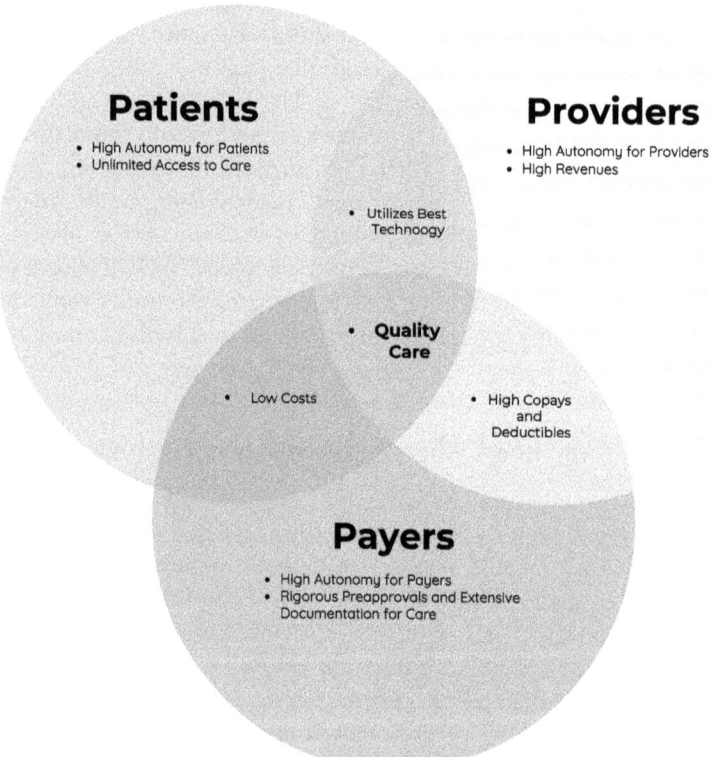

Figure 3.1 Misaligned incentives in US health care

payers. Unfortunately, but not surprisingly, the motivations of these key players do not always overlap, and they are incentivized by different goals/objectives. Here are three observations in this regard. First, the most consequential misalignment is regarding costs. Patients and payers are generally motivated to decrease health care expenditures, which they call "costs." Providers are generally motivated to increase health care expenditures, which they call "revenues." This is a reflection of the business bromide that one entity's costs are another entity's revenues. Second, the major actors want substantial autonomy. Patients want to be able to access any physician or health care network at any time and at low/no cost. Providers want autonomy to practice medicine and administer health care according to their own best judgment, without undue influence from payers or regulators. Payers want to be able to deny coverage either before or after care, as well as set the reimbursement rates. However, the system cannot function effectively if everyone were to have autonomy, assuming that is even possible. Third, there is one goal that patients, providers, and payers agree on: quality. Albeit for slightly different reasons, all three are motivated to improve the quality of patient outcomes, and that commonality represents common ground to build upon.

Overutilization is a particularly vivid way in which one sees the adverse incentives playing out. About 80 percent of health care dollars are spent on 20 percent of the population, some of whom have a legitimate need for above-average health expenditure but many of whom are over-consumptive. Are high-deductible plans efficient as a way to discourage excessive use by patients? In theory, having a high deductible is a smart way to de-incentivize patients from seeking too much care. It has the potential to remove the moral hazard where a person naturally tends to overconsume a product or service that they are not paying for directly. For example, imagine that there is no copay and no deductible. One is reminded of the classic case of the patient who visits the emergency room seeking treatment for the common cold. Now, imagine a different person, with a cold, who has to personally pay for that emergency room visit. Presumably, they would rest at home, drink plenty of liquids, and take relatively inexpensive **over-the-counter medicines.**

However, a potential danger in high-deductible plans is that they may discourage the preventive care that can diagnose and treat health problems before they grow more expensive. In some cases, this proactive care can prevent a problem from developing at all. Since patients with a high-deductible plan often forgo their preventative care, high-deductible plans can end up costing more in the long run. Health plans fully recognize this duality, so many try to "split the difference" by having relatively high copays and deductibles for nonpreventative care but having the patient incur very little or even zero cost for pursuing preventative care.

Emergency departments (EDs) in the United States tend to be extraordinarily expensive. This gives rise to another interesting and odd duality regarding EDs. On the one hand, because hospital emergency rooms are so expensive, many patients who are medically justified forgo treatment, leading to a worsening condition or even death. On the other hand, because EDs are generally so accessible (e.g., open 24/7 and always fully staffed), many other patients seek the immediacy of emergency care, even when it is medically unnecessary. Thus, EDs are often both simultaneously underused and overused.

What's the answer? It's twofold, designed to address this dual problem caused by misaligned incentives. First, it is essential to make emergency care more affordable so high-acuity cases are in no way dissuaded from seeking out these services. Second, we need to make communities and the general public aware of the availability of less costly care facilities. In general, there needs to be increased education about the differences between primary care facilities, urgent care facilities, and emergency rooms, so patients can find the right fit depending on their symptoms.

Relative to peer nations, the US federal and state governments are considerably more hands-off when it comes to cost containment, efficiency maximization, and incentive alignment. This might seem like a good thing, given the normal inefficiency of large government bureaucracies. In health care, there is a misconception that the private sector is necessarily more efficient than the public sector. This is not always the case. For example, private insurance administrative costs are estimated to often exceed 15 percent, but Medicare's administrative costs are often less than 5 percent.[4] Thus, government can play a pro-efficiency role, especially in realigning incentives to yield more effective/efficient outcomes.

3.2 Cost as a Primary Barrier

High out-of-pocket (OOP) costs (e.g., copays, deductibles), even for patients with insurance, are a substantial barrier to accessing health care. Nearly one-third of Americans say that high OOP health care costs create a challenge to treatment.[5] Worse yet, in any given year, approximately 27 percent of US adults actually do skip some form of medical services

[4] Archer, "Medicare Is More Efficient."   [5] Gallup, "Healthcare Affordability and Value."

(e.g., tests, treatments, visits, or prescription fills) because of the financial burden.[6] For the uninsured, this number rises to over 69 percent.[7] People are often forced to choose between buying food, paying the rent, or covering health care costs. Given this choice, good mental and physical health often gets sacrificed. Unfortunately, there is a trend toward – not away from – deductible plans that are equivalent to having no insurance at all, except in the most catastrophic situations. Americans facing these high costs in copays, **coinsurances**, and deductibles routinely face Hobbesian choices.

Most insured American adults are actively concerned about their ability to pay monthly health **insurance premiums**. Moreover, even large percentages of adults with employer-sponsored insurance or marketplace coverage rate their insurance as being "fair" or "poor" regarding the level of monthly premiums and the OOP costs for utilization.[8] Furthermore, health care debt is a massive burden for a significant share of Americans. Over 40 percent say they are concerned with debts owed to banks, credit cards, family/friends, and other lenders that are attributable to medical or dental expenses. Sadly, this also disproportionately affects certain groups: Blacks and Hispanics, low-income adults, parents, uninsured adults, and women.[9]

A sizable proportion of the US population lives just one accident or illness away from financial ruin and personal bankruptcy. There are three main reasons why those who are hardworking and employed still lack health care coverage: (i) it is not offered by employer (e.g., use of independent contractor status rather than paying as a normal, full-time W2), (ii) the cost of the insurance is too high (e.g., excessively high deductibles and premiums could cause an otherwise eligible employee to decline coverage), and (iii) the employee is not eligible (e.g., does not work enough hours per week). Many of the uninsured are employed individuals, dependents of the employed, or dependents of unemployed. These are sympathetic cases. Government initiatives designed to help uninsured individuals secure health care coverage through state and federal programs are helpful in lessening the impact of uninsured status as a barrier to health care coverage.

Many Americans are left to the absolutely worst-case scenario: no insurance. The OOP model involves patients having to pay for their medical products and services themselves, sometimes taking cash or

---

[6] Board of Governors of the Federal Reserve System, *Well-Being of U.S. Households*.
[7] Lopes et al., "Healthcare Costs." [8] Lopes et al., "Healthcare Costs."
[9] Lopes et al., "Healthcare Costs."

other forms of payment (e.g., check) literally from their pockets, paying directly, without any subsequent reimbursement or insurance coverage. The OOP approach is commonly found in less developed areas and countries. Many countries in Africa, Asia, and South America, as well as regions in the United States, with large uninsured or underinsured populations, have widespread OOP. Leaving Americans to an OOP model for their health care costs subjects them unnecessarily to a type of financial Russian roulette.

3.3 Access as a Secondary Barrier

In addition to affordability, accessibility is the second-most significant barrier in the US health care system. Access can be measured at different units of analysis: block group, census tract, zip code, county, congressional district, metro division, metro area, and state. The physical availability of health care is usually defined as the geographic proximity of facilities and providers in relation to communities and individuals; it represents the ability of the medical service market to effectively meet the health needs of the local population. In the United States, nearly 85 million people live in areas with a shortage of primary care health professionals.[10] There are **medically underserved areas/populations** and **health professional shortage areas**. There are also pharmacy deserts, and over 40 million Americans live in these areas, making it more challenging to fill prescriptions.[11]

Care starts with having a health care professional, principally a physician, available to administer said services. However, no health care provider generally means no health care provision, and this is the sad situation facing many areas and regions of the United States. The number of medical schools and the number of training spots available to new doctors have both been held relatively constant in the United States. Perhaps with good reason because of the typically high annual incomes physicians can eventually make, the higher education system in the US puts the burden of financing largely on students, who are usually forced to borrow substantial sums given the relatively more expensive cost of American medical schools. The debt load upon graduation incentivizes many new physicians to pursue more lucrative specialty practice areas rather than work in family medicine and primary care. Thus, the US

[10] KFF, "Health Professional Shortage Areas."   [11] Pennic, "Healthcare Deserts."

physician shortage is partially attributable to high rates of specialization and the way in which medical education is structured.

Generally speaking, urban areas have a high density of physicians, but even within cities, the primary care physician (PCP) shortage can impact low-income populations and Medicaid enrollees, especially those also living in underserved neighborhoods. Many private practices operating in underserved areas struggle financially. They will often end up completely relocating to less economically poor neighborhoods or deciding to limit the number of patients who use Medicaid as well as patients who are uninsured and underinsured. The physician gap is particularly acute in the mental health arena. The United States has a mere 0.14 psychiatrists per 1,000 residents, coming in as the second lowest of all peer nations; only 6 percent of US-trained medical school graduates enter psychiatry. One key reason is that psychiatrists, despite the increasing demand for mental health service, remain one of the lowest-paid physician specialties in the United States.[12] In addition to physicians, there are shortages of nurses, community health workers (CHWs), pharmacists, paramedics, and physical/occupational therapists. One key issue, especially during and subsequent to the COVID-19 epidemic, was health care professionals experiencing mental and physical exhaustion. Implementing team-based care using care coordination and performance-based bonuses can help reduce provider burnout rates.

Nowhere is the shortage of health care workers more dire than in the rural part of the United States. Over 45 million Americans live in rural areas.[13] A disproportionate number of rural residents either depend on Medicaid or they lack insurance coverage. Approximately one-third of veterans enrolled in the Veterans Health Administration (VHA) live in rural locations. The VHA has an Office of Rural Health that is responsible for supporting initiatives and researching issues that impact rural veterans. Tragically, rural communities experience higher rates of maternal mortality and other negative health outcomes.

Why is that? Rural communities often lack large hospital systems. Moreover, the well-off populations, who would normally be able to pay for services, as well as providers, especially physicians and nurses, are often unwilling to be based in these locations. This creates shortages, meaning that people often have to travel long distances for care. A study in *The Journal of Rural Health* found that cancer patients in rural areas traveled an

---

[12] U.S. Bureau of Labor Statistics, *Occupational Employment and Wages*.
[13] U.S. Department of Agriculture, *ERS Charts of Note*.

average of 41 miles to get radiation treatment.[14] And if this is the average, there will be many patients needing to travel well over 50 miles for these life-preserving services. Traveling these long distances takes time (often time away from work) and can be expensive.

Over 80 percent of rural patients live in counties labeled by the federal government as medically underserved (e.g., one physician within an 11,000-square-mile area). In recent years, financial stresses have caused many rural hospitals to shut down,[15] with over 5 percent in the last decade.[16] Over half of rural counties in the United States have no hospital-based obstetric services. From a workforce development perspective, we need to increase the education and training opportunities for health care professionals who are considering working in rural areas. Indian Health Service reports sizeable vacancy rates for clinical providers in areas that provide direct care to AI/AN people, which has a deleterious impact on patient access, care quality, and employee morale. Rural communities continue to have fewer broadband internet options than urban ones, which often limits the applicability of telehealth. Compared to only 1.5 percent in urban areas, 22.3 percent of those in rural areas lack broadband internet access.[17]

3.4 Nonhealth Determinants of Health

Many Americans face barriers to care that are not of their own making. Barriers to accessing care include costs, geography, and transportation. Another more hidden barrier is the real and perceived lack of fair treatment and respect that potential health care users experience from provider institutions and individuals. For example, language barriers often make it challenging for patients to understand what health services are available and then to effectively communicate with an organization's staff. Patients with limited English proficiency tend to experience increased medical errors, lengthier hospital stays, and greater rates of readmission.[18] Translation services should be available, as needed, for areas with multilingual populations. Cultural competency training for providers can help reduce language barriers. Additionally, stigmas around mental health,

---

[14] Longacre et al., "Evaluating Travel Distance."
[15] American Hospital Association, "AHA Report."
[16] Center for Healthcare Quality and Payment Reform, "Rural Healthcare."
[17] U.S. Department of Agriculture, *Broadband*.
[18] Agency for Healthcare Research and Quality, *Executive Summary*.

substance use, and reproductive health can prevent individuals from disclosing relevant issues to their care provider.

The social drivers of health (SDOH) – also called social determinants of health – impinge directly on health care access.[19] Why? How? Because where a patient is born, lives, learns, plays, prays, and works impacts a wide range of quality-of-life outcomes. The built environment is part of the SDOH, which focuses on the community- and neighborhood-level factors. **Health-related social needs (HRSN)** are cultural, economic, and social needs that impact an individual's experience and affect their ability to improve their health and well-being.[20] These needs include access to affordable/stable housing, financial stability, healthy food, health care, and transportation. People who live in HRSN areas also tend to experience higher levels of air pollution, making them considerably more likely to develop respiratory conditions such as asthma, chronic obstructive pulmonary disease, and emphysema.[21] Patients lacking affordable and reliable transportation often struggle to keep medical appointments. SDOH and HRSN typically intersect. For example, in terms of HRSN, a patient may earn below the federal poverty line, and in terms of SDOH, they also live in an area with substandard economic conditions. People residing in "food deserts" face significant challenges achieving a nutritious diet, which increases the risk of severe conditions such as diabetes, heart disease, and obesity.

Steps the government can take: screen for HRSN, provide referrals to community resources, provide referrals to regional social services, and provide professionals (e.g., care navigators, CHWs, social workers) who can help patients. An effective screening assessment for HRSN should ask questions regarding family and community support, education, employment, financial strain, food security, living situation, safety, transportation, and utilities. The government cannot mandate that providers show caring and warmth per se, but it can encourage and incentivize providers to create environments that are conducive to good care. In this way, some health disparities are eminently preventable. Health equity is the highest state achievable where all patients have a fair and just opportunity to become their healthiest self regardless of disability, race, ethnicity, gender identity, geography, sexual orientation, preferred language, or socioeconomic status negatively affecting their access to care and, ultimately, affecting the

---

[19] U.S. Department of Health and Human Services, *Healthy People 2030*.
[20] Centers for Medicare and Medicaid Services, *Health Related Social Needs*.
[21] Duan, Hao, and Yang, "Air Pollution."

outcome.[22] Not surprisingly, barriers to care contribute substantially to disparities and poor outcomes. Prospective patients will avoid medical care if they believe there is likely to be disrespect or mistreatment.

Continuing to think about other potential barriers, internet access is increasingly seen as a "super determinant" because of the direct role it can play in accessing telehealth and by influencing other social determinants such as education and employment. The internet has now become an essential element of daily life, including health and wellness. Yet, high-speed internet use rates tend to be considerably lower in households where the primary occupant is sixty-five years or older, has a disability, has low income, is in a rural location, or is Hispanic, African American, American Indian, or Alaskan Native.[23] In the health care context, the digital divide is sometimes called the "broadband health gap."[24] The nation's digital divide reflects and then deepens inequities in terms of who can and cannot access high-speed internet. The strong connection between broadband access and health care outcomes is ever more closely linking digital equity and health equity. Federal, state, and local governments are helping stimulate public–private conversations about digital exclusion and equitable utilization of telehealth services. Major projects underway to expand internet access include: Capital Projects Fund, FCC Affordable Connectivity Plan, FCC National Broadband Map, Internet for All, Lifeline, Mapping Broadband Health in America, and ReConnect Loan and Grant Program. Despite all these projects, the effort to make sure all counties have broadband access remains a work in progress.

3.5 Mobile Clinics, School-Based Health Centers, and Telehealth

Innovative alternative care settings have emerged to help patients without a regular PCP attain improved health outcomes, lower overall health care costs, experience fewer hospitalizations, lower the likelihood of treatment duplication, and lessen the prevalence of disparities.[25] Federally Qualified Health Center (FQHC) offers neighborhood clinics that can provide basic primary care. Without access to caring, comforting health providers, patients often suffer through undue pain and their conditions may worsen over time, becoming much more complex and expensive to treat. Safety net providers like FQHC focus on providing critical care to the poor, the

---

[22] Centers for Medicare and Medicaid Services, *Health Equity*.
[23] American Health Information Management Association Foundation, "Health Equity."
[24] Federal Communications Commission, *Advancing Broadband Connectivity*.
[25] Savoy, Hazlett-O'Brien, and Rapacciuolo, "Primary Care Physicians."

uninsured, the underinsured, Medicaid recipients, and other vulnerable patients. Because of chronic underinvestment in the United States, public transit in many areas is unreliable and sometimes even too costly for many low-income patients. And unfortunately, nonemergency medical transportation, as well as ride-sharing services such as Lyft and Uber, are often inconvenient and unreliable for patients.

We discussed transportation issues in the context of rural areas, but mobility challenges can also impact those living in urban and suburban regions. It is a ubiquitous problem. Therefore, US health care providers are increasingly investing in innovative alternative treatment sites. Mobile clinics are a popular tool for serving health care deserts in rural and urban areas. For example, instead of making patients take a time-consuming and potentially expensive trip to a clinic or hospital, many providers are now offering mobile clinics that come right to where people live and work. Essentially, the institution comes to the patient rather than the patient going to the institution. During COVID-19, when the ability to congregate in public facilities like hospitals was limited, many health care providers offered buses, trailers, and vans providing pandemic testing and treatment, while also including other basic medical services (e.g., blood pressure check). In some cases, a fast-food-restaurant-style, drive-up service was offered so that people could even remain inside their vehicles. Many communities have smartly repurposed mobile vans, previously launched to provide testing and vaccinations during the COVID-19 pandemic, to provide a breadth of primary care services.

School-based health centers (SBHCs) are, as the name suggests, entities offering physically embedded medical services. The target population is of course children, and they provide K–12 students with access to primary care, which can increase both health and educational outcomes. Unfortunately, only about 10 percent of public schools contain an SBHC. Another innovative approach is to have free-standing EDs. This can provide acute/urgent care for communities that otherwise lack a hospital. To fully leverage these mobile solutions and other alternative sites so that they can be better staffed, state and local governments should relax restrictions on nurse practitioners and physician assistants, allowing them to practice independently.

Telehealth (also called telemedicine or virtual health care) leverages cloud-based data and videoconferencing to allow health care professionals to reach large and distant geographies. Telehealth can be used as a workaround to some transportation challenges. By eliminating the need to travel to a doctor for routine checks, patients are empowered to connect for remote checkups. Telehealth also enables small-town physicians to connect their patients with specialists and coordinate holistic care that is better overall. Once the initial infrastructure investment is made in telehealth, the marginal cost of using the system itself is relatively low. Audio-only telehealth visits remove the need for a smartphone or broadband internet. Some older patients are resistant to telehealth, but it is clearly here to stay and will be expanding.

3.6 Universal Health Care and Other Government Solutions

Universal health coverage (UHC) involves all people having full access to quality health care services when/where it is needed and without financial hardship. In terms of etymology, *universal* means "everyone." The universality should capture the full continuum of health services, including education, prevention, diagnoses, treatment, rehabilitation, and palliative care. Every country has its own pathway to attaining and maintaining UHC. Most countries have hybrid models for achieving it. In the second part of the twentieth century, European countries all gradually adopted universal health care to cover almost all citizens. There is no single European health care system, and social protection is not under the jurisdiction of the European Commission. Thus, given that it is the authority of individual national governments, each country has its own, slightly different, system. In Europe, the provision of UHC ranges from government-owned health facilities to highly regulated compulsory insurance schemes, but in most countries, the funding for universal health care coverage comes from taxes.

At some level, UHC is fundamentally a political issue and is part of an ongoing debate about the role of government in our lives. Many argue that UHC is a fundamental human right[26] and believe that employment should not determine access to health care. There are pros and cons of universal health care. Potential advantages for countries and covered lives include: greater price transparency, enhanced health care equity/parity, increased life expectancy in the population, and lower overall health care costs. For sure, a free-at-point-of-use health care system can lower administrative burdens. Yet, some argue that potential disadvantages include: healthy people have to pay for the services of unhealthy people, the relatively well-off financially have to pay for the medical services of the relatively poor, it requires careful public management, it has the potential to increase fiscal

---

[26] Ranabhat et al., "Universal Health Coverage Evolution."

3.6 Universal Health Care and Government Solutions

pressures, and it can make access to medical services more challenging. When there is a single-payer government system with a low cost and a standard benefit, there can be overutilization, which then requires having regulations in place to manage demand. The potential for a long waitlist and delays in treatment are often offered as additional potential downsides of a national health insurance model.

UHC programs provide essential services such as health promotion, preventive health, diagnosis, medical treatment, rehabilitation, palliative care, and hospice care. The types of potential universal health care systems include the full mix: public provider and public payer, public provider and private payer, private provider and public payer, or private provider and private payer. Done properly, UHC can expand access and empower patients, their families, and their caregivers to build lasting, meaningful relationships with specific health care providers and even medical institutions. This creates stronger, healthier, and more economically prosperous communities. Education, as part of universal coverage, is another means of empowerment. Personal health literacy measures the extent to which individuals can find, understand, and consume information and services to inform health-related decisions and actions. Many Americans lack basic health literacy, which is disempowering. **Community health workers** can be great resources for education and empowerment. Unfortunately, it has been a challenge in some states to create stable funding streams to support CHWs. They are often paid through grants, which is typically not a stable source. To address this, some states are allowing CHWs to bill Medicaid. Making their services reimbursable could help support this workforce and some states are starting to do this.

A public health orientation is a key underpinning of any successful governmental approach to health care, whether universal or not. Patient-based approaches address the needs of individuals. Public health addresses the needs of the broader community. Governments generally gain a strong ROI with investments in public health. In particular, early prevention is relatively inexpensive yet can prevent or at least ameliorate dire and expensive health problems. Elements of an effective public health system include robust communication, strong data analysis and utilization, comprehensive planning, community mobilization, extensive collaboration/partnering, analysis and decision support, research, evaluation, and quality improvement. Enhancing the public health infrastructure is a key part of reducing chronic diseases and being proactive regarding future health crises. For example, access to preventive care and treatment is crucial for cardiovascular health. Research shows that by improving health care access, population-level cardiovascular disease risk may be reduced.

With regard to advancing universal health care access, data is key. Not having a detailed understanding of where care is lacking, why, and for whom makes it considerably more challenging for government entities to design and implement solutions. Governments need to take an active role in compiling and analyzing data about everything from patient demographics to service providers and insurance coverage. Key information includes chronic condition diagnoses, health insurance coverage, health-linked behaviors such as exercise/nutrition, mental health, preventive health screenings, and substance use. Government also needs to understand benchmarks and keep up with the latest trends in uninsurance patterns/rates.

Ultimately, to address insurance gaps, for instance, governments can increase funding for Medicaid and the Children's Health Insurance Program, which serve to broaden health care coverage for low-income individuals and families. Raising the reimbursement rates and reducing the administrative burden related to these programs would make them considerably less difficult for health care providers to accept. Many eligible low-income Americans find it complicated and cumbersome to enroll in subsidized insurance or Medicaid. Federal and state governments could make that considerably easier, including minimizing the bureaucratic barriers to Medicaid eligibility determinations. Technology, including artificial intelligence, deep learning, and machine learning, offers the potential to improve the administrative efficiency related to payments.

Chapter Summary

This chapter builds off the previous chapter by taking a balanced approach to the federal government's involvement in health care by recognizing its potential concerns as well as the value it can bring. The two primary challenges for the US health care system to tackle are access and affordability. We focus particularly on the key metric of access to health care, with international comparisons and examples provided to highlight the value of a universal health care option as a way of ensuring that all members in a society can utilize health care. We closed by positing the need for balanced coverage options. In health care, an iron law prevails: One person/entity's costs are another person/entity's revenues. This makes change difficult, being that it is economically and politically fraught, so transitioning to an extreme one-provider, one-payer form of universal health care in the United States would be enormously difficult. Fortunately, there are multiple types of universal systems, and there are a slew of creative micro-solutions that can be implemented, regardless of universality.

CHAPTER 4

Private Industry as a Partner in Health Care

Insights

- Moving first toward essential packages of health services (EPHS) is an excellent incremental way to achieve universal health care coverage (UHC).
- The private sector also includes the not-for-profit and NGO sectors.
- There is a trend for private health insurance companies to be more involved with public insurance programs.
- The private sector is even more diverse and heterogeneous than the public sector.
- We have to distinguish between "good" innovation and "bad" innovation in health care; sometimes innovators can destroy value more rapidly than they create it.

Health Care systems worldwide grapple with the challenge of delivering quality, accessible, and equitable care to diverse populations. At the heart of this endeavor lies the interplay between public and private health insurance models. Public health insurance, often managed by government entities and funded through taxation, aims to provide universal coverage, ensuring that financial constraints do not bar individuals from receiving essential health care. Conversely, private health insurance, offered by commercial entities, emphasizes flexibility and customization, allowing individuals to tailor coverage to their specific needs.

While both systems have inherent strengths and limitations, their integration through public–private partnerships (PPPs) presents a compelling solution to fill the gaps that neither sector can address alone. Public–private partnerships, as structured collaborations between public institutions and private entities, have been instrumental in addressing health care access challenges, especially in resource-limited settings. By leveraging the innovation and operational efficiency of the private sector alongside the public sector's focus on equity and community welfare, such partnerships can unlock significant opportunities for improved health care delivery.

A **PPP** is an agreement between one or more public entities and one or more private entities, working in a mutually beneficial, structured relationship, and often on a medium- to longer-term basis. This chapter examines the dynamic interaction between public and private health insurance, the role of PPPs in addressing systemic challenges, and the pathways to fostering synergies between these sectors to achieve universal health coverage. By delving into the complexities of these models, we explore how innovative collaborations can redefine the future of health care, ensuring that quality care is accessible to all.

Private health insurance, as the name suggests, is offered by private companies, allowing individuals to choose plans according to their specific preferences and requirements. In contrast, public health insurance is usually owned and operated (or subsidized) by a governmental entity with the objective of providing coverage to all citizens, regardless of their ability to pay; however, care and coverage options are less customizable. Public health insurance is usually a statutory entitlement provided by a governmental entity. "Public" coverage means government health insurance programs paid for by taxpayers, whereas "private" generally means commercial insurance coverage paid for by employers and individuals. Often called universal insurance, this public health care is managed by government agencies and/or highly regulated private-sector providers.

4.1 Public–Private Partnerships

Relying solely on the public sector to provide primary health care services in low- and middle-income countries can have limitations, including a shortage of health care professionals, inefficient institutional frameworks, inadequate quality, and suboptimal efficiency. This is especially true for remote and rural areas. To address this, many have suggested expanding PPPs for the provision of health services in these countries.[1] In the hospital context, studies find that PPPs can yield favorable outcomes in terms of effectiveness and efficiency.[2] A similar logic can be applied to the United States, particularly in certain regions. Collaboration with the private sector is essential to reaching public health system goals, especially universal coverage. And what do private-sector entities have to gain? The benefits include increasing revenue, opening new markets, building goodwill,

---

[1] Joudyian et al., "Public-Private Partnerships."   [2] Rodrigues, "Public-Private Partnerships."

strengthening reputation, and contributing to overall community/population health.

Public–private partnerships are common in the nonhealth care sectors of the economy (e.g., energy, education, infrastructure, transportation). The PPP model can allow federal, state, and local governments to attract financial and technical capabilities. At least theoretically, PPPs are a classic win–win opportunity. PPPs can enhance performance, cost-effectiveness, risk allocation, and service delivery, allowing government to access new sources of funding, especially during conditions of budgetary constraints. A well-designed and executed PPP should combine the strengths of private partners (e.g., entrepreneurship, innovation, management efficiency, and technological savviness) with the strengths of public partners (e.g., emphasis on equity/justice, local knowledge, public accountability, and social responsibility).

The private and public sectors should operate in a complementary manner, and private providers should not operate in isolation. Since *private health providers (PHPs)* are a component of the mixed US health system, they need to complement the public sector and not operate in isolation or opposition. Broad guidelines for effective public–private collaboration include: (i) creating mutual value, (ii) setting out the goals and expectations of both types of entities, (iii) clearly identifying the comparative strengths and limitations, (iv) determining the comparative advantages of each sector performing any given service, (v) maintaining a bidirectional flow of data and information, and (vi) building trust in the population being served.[3] Another increasingly important enabler for collaboration is the application of analytics, artificial intelligence, and machine learning to help solve complex problems.

The parties to a PPP typically share costs, benefits, resources, risks, and responsibilities, so determining strategic capability and aligning each party's goals are crucial. There are many risks in any health care contract, including financial, logistical, medical, procurement, supply, and technological. There should be equitable risk-sharing and effective dispute resolution. In the typical PPP, the private-sector entities take on significant financial, operational, and technical risks while the public entities are held accountable for defined outcomes (e.g., they take on the political risk). Trust between the sectors is built through discussion, negotiation, and ongoing interaction over time. Governments should develop public–private dialogue platforms, so the exchange of best practices is institutionalized rather than limited to

---

[3] Arnaout et al., "Technology in Public-Private Partnerships."

isolated one-offs. For their part, private health care providers should consider how they can prepare to work more effectively with the public sector to achieve universal health coverage and other key goals.

Government health systems are facing growing pressure as they struggle to satisfy universal health coverage goals. To reach universal coverage goals globally by 2030, it would take an estimated 25,000 new hospitals, 350,000 new clinics, and over 20 million additional health workers.[4] Moreover, from 2026 to 2039, an investment of about $370 billion would be needed per year, for a total of well over $1 trillion.[5] However, this investment would save an estimated 100 million lives by 2030.[6] From a social determinants of health perspective, removing as many health deserts as possible is another laudatory goal. The World Health Organization recommends that everyone live within about a 5-km (or about 3.1 miles) radius of a health facility for optimal access to health care.[7] In addition to availability, we also have to be attentive to quality, for example by reducing episodes of iatrogenesis, which refers to the unintentional effects or complications resulting from medical errors (advice, diagnosis, or treatment).

Essential packages of health services are the core health care services that should be readily available and affordable through the public, private, or NGO sectors, including a hybrid system.[8] Examples of EPHS include annual physical exams, vaccinations, and preventative diagnostic tests. Mental health is a significant area where insurance coverage gaps need to be filled. One way to progressively move toward UHC is to adopt EPHS. This is where the private sector can play a significant role in regard to health care, and the key here is PPPs. For example, the government may be able to help with large-scale, strategic purchasing while private-sector actors do the implementation of new services.

The COVID-19 crisis offers some examples of collaborative public/private/NGO partnerships. During the COVID-19 pandemic, when health systems faced unprecedented demands, the need for public–private collaboration in health care came to the forefront. The private sector generally rose to the occasion and provided crucial COVID-19 testing and treatment for many patients. This included the extremely sick, who required treatment in intensive care units, particularly in certain pockets of the United States, where local public health systems faced severe constraints in capacity, know-how, and resources for coping with the crisis.

---

[4] World Health Organization, "Global Health Targets."
[5] Stenberg et al., "Financing Transformative Health Systems."
[6] World Health Organization, "Global Health Targets." [7] Weiss et al., "Maps of Travel Time."
[8] Wright and Holtz, "Essential Packages."

The COVID-19 pandemic vividly demonstrated that private-sector expertise, knowledge, and other resources can be leveraged to improve and expand the delivery of health-related goods and services, including a broader role in the maintenance of essential services and in ensuring system resilience.[9]

Public–private partnerships are not miracle solutions, so continual assessment of their efficacy is warranted. To facilitate comparative evaluation, we have to use empirical benchmarking to find solutions in health care. When evaluating the private sector, we can take one of three approaches to evaluation. First, we can compare it to how the public sector would perform. Second, we can examine it in isolation. Third, we can compare it to an optimized collaboration with the public sector. The third approach is best, and we should employ it frequently to assess how any given PPP is performing.

4.2 Leveraging the Private Sector in Health Care

Public–private partnerships are powerful tools for potentially extending public health's reach to improve/save lives in the workplace and at home, accelerating innovation, and changing the way government conceptualizes and solves problems. There are opportunities for formal and informal collaborations leading to valuable mutual benefits. Collaboration is particularly valuable when challenges are complex and ill-defined like securing universal health coverage. Universal health care coverage around the world is financed and delivered by the public sector, but the potential contributions of the private health sector remain untapped.[10] There is a tremendous opportunity for the private health sector to become major actors in the attainment of universal health coverage. Public–private partnerships can help governmental entities improve performance by doing more with less, building on the capabilities of others, leveraging collective action, and realizing cost savings.

Increased private contracting in health services would be an efficient and logical step, moving further toward providing more accessible, affordable, and sustainable health care for all. Collaborating with the private sector can help federal, state, and local governments that are coping with lower-income regions reduce existing gaps in health services, better leverage the considerable private data, knowledge, and technology, and shift some of the burden

---

[9] Maresso et al., "Engaging the Private Sector."
[10] World Health Organization, "Universal Health Coverage."

of health care investment from public taxpayers to private investors. For example, private-sector providers can help with the active redirection from emergency departments to physician offices and **urgent care clinics**. Involvement of the private sector can also be used to enable existing infrastructure to be used more efficiently. In these ways, we can harness the private sector for collaboration on attaining universal health coverage.[11]

Typically, the private sector is flexible and nimble, and it can be used to counterbalance the bureaucracy and slow pace of the public sector. Private entities (e.g., angel investors, family offices, private equity, venture capital) can also bring new sources of capital and investment. Private equity has funded many new companies focused on cutting costs (via increasing efficiencies), enhancing revenue (via increasing prices or utilization), and, most importantly, improving quality (via better devices, diagnostics, drugs, and procedures). The basic business model underlying many private sector–funded actors is developing innovations that meaningfully impact access, affordability, and quality for patients, families, and communities. Many startup companies have grown rapidly and have achieved success with this model, even garnering exits at exceptionally high valuations (e.g., Iora Health, Oak Street Health, One Medical, Summit Health-CityMD, and VillageMD).

To properly leverage the private sector, we have to understand the complexity and diversity of private health ecosystems. The heterogeneity of private-sector actors can make it difficult to grasp the full scope of their potential contributions to UHC. The private sector includes entrepreneurs – small, medium, and large – and conglomerate companies. Additionally, the private health sector includes both for-profit and not-for-profit social entities. We can make a distinction between for-profit private organizations and not-for-profit private organizations based, as the names suggest, on whether the primary mandate is to make profits or to serve broader societal interests. And even within the social sector, there is a mix of faith-based organizations (e.g., churches), NGOs (e.g., World Health Organization), humanitarian-oriented not-for-profit organizations (e.g., American Cancer Society, American Heart Association), and professional membership organizations (e.g., American Medical Association). And of course, in the United States, many large, prominent, highly profitable providers (e.g., Advocate Health, Ascension Health, CommonSpirit Health, and Trinity Health) and payers (e.g., Blue Cross/Blue Shield companies, Geisinger, and Kaiser Permanente) are formally structured as not-for-profit organizations.

[11] Clarke, "Harnessing Private Sector Collaboration."

The primary mandate for any CEO leading a for-profit, private-sector organization is to maximize profits within the bounds of ethical and legal conduct. Those leaders have a legally binding duty of care and duty of loyalty to the corporation. However, this itself has advantages and disadvantages for public health and society more broadly. Private health entities operate with profit as their primary objective and are highly market-oriented. Private-sector providers require clear and compelling financial incentives, and they are designed to be more responsive to market demand and supply dynamics. Another expectation of mixed markets is that they can improve quality by increasing competition between the public and private sectors.

Governments frequently ask (and sometimes essentially require) private contractors to provide services at unprofitable price points, and those losses usually cannot be made up on volume. Doing higher volume at unfavorable prices is just a prescription for losing money faster. To the extent possible, government has to strive for the private-sector provider to be aligned with public-sector goals including universal health coverage. Without any public subsidy, the private sector – as the profit maximizer it should be – generally provides only a limited set of services and some public health services may be neglected. Quality can suffer when the primary focus is on maximizing profits rather than on patient care per se. The counterargument is that financial accountability and the profit motive incentivize private companies to maximize patients' well-being, be innovative, and eliminate unneeded bureaucracy.

In health care, services are often provided that are valuable, but not very profitable. There have been some privately owned hospitals that failed (i.e., closed and/or went bankrupt), in large part because they were serving high percentages of low-income or uninsured patients. Not every health care business deserves to survive, and when a business fails that deserves to fail (e.g., because it persistently offered low quality at unreasonable prices), resources are freed up that can then flow to higher-value enterprises. Organizational failure happens in all sectors, but health care is fundamentally different because closure is so costly to communities, families, and patients. Thus, one downside of greater reliance on the private sector is this potentiality of closure.

4.3 Advantages and Disadvantages of the Public and Private Sector

It is useful to consider in more detail the advantages and disadvantages of the public sector, as well as the advantages and disadvantages of the private sector. Public health insurance generally has the following positive attributes: universal access (e.g., every individual has coverage regardless of their financial circumstances), cost-effectiveness (achieved primarily via large economies of scale and scope), and a heavy focus on preventive care (e.g., vaccinations). For routine and simple ailments, the public sector may be more efficient in controlling overuse of resources and treatments, as well as providing preventive and public health services.[12]

Public health insurance generally has the following negatives: limited choice (i.e., potential restricted availability of providers and treatments), longer waiting times (i.e., given high demand and limited supply, there can be extended waits), and government influence/interference (i.e., political decisions can impact coverage). Public health care plans often offer fewer options for health services than private health care plans, which makes it easier for the latter's policyholders to access needed care. Sometimes public health care recipients need to wait for medical treatment because the system prioritizes patients who require urgent attention. An extended wait can cause increased suffering, worsened symptoms, more expensive care, and a longer recovery. From broader organizational and structural perspectives, the public sector is often constrained by functional silos, partisan politics, rigid cultures, strict regulations, and few incentives. All of these tend to stifle innovation.

The private sector can contribute considerable expertise and resources, so failing to fully use them means governments miss potential health improvement opportunities. Private health insurance generally has the following positive attributes: comprehensive coverage (e.g., elective treatments, specialized care), customizable coverage (e.g., choosing the level of copay and deductible), and faster access to care (i.e., shorter wait times for appointments and procedures). As a result of these generally shorter service waiting times, private health care insurance policyholders typically have faster access to needed care and thus potentially fewer long-term repercussions. Looking at the bigger picture, the private sector can help improve quality of care through increased market competition along with the benefits of being more flexible and consumer-centered.

Even in countries where public health care is available, people sometimes prefer private health care. There are usually three primary reasons: (i) access, (ii) coverage, and (iii) quality. This trend is likely to continue with the preferences of the younger generation. A study from the UK shows that, relative to older people, younger people (between eighteen and thirty-

---

[12] Morgan, Ensor, and Waters, "Private Sector Healthcare."

four years of age) are usually more: positive about private-sector services, willing to use them, likely to have used them, and likely to have paid for their own treatment.[13] In the United States, young adults have grown up in a world with health apps, telehealth, retail clinics, and urgent care clinics, as well as the overall system being mixed-mode. Accordingly, there are likely to be more fluid and flexible views regarding the relationship between public and private health care.

Private health providers are no more a panacea for the problems of the US health care system than is the government. Private health insurance generally has the following negatives: higher costs, potential preexisting conditions barrier, limitations on some more expensive treatments, and potential for profit-driven rather than public health–oriented decision-making. Private health services do hold the potential to increase the overall costs of care via overuse (e.g., ordering diagnostic services and prescribing expensive medications).

4.4 Mixed Systems in US Health Care

The various national contexts in which UHC would be implemented are diverse and are usually not amenable to standardized approaches. Moreover, most health care systems are not configured in a carefully planned way. They are more unintended than intended. The United States has a hybrid system consisting of private health insurance provided by employers, health care exchanges, public plans, and out-of-pocket self-pay. The private health care sector can be highly differentiated, insufficiently documented, and unevenly regulated, so it is considerably more heterogeneous than the public sector.

There are three prominent frameworks used to provide universal health care. They are worth covering in more detail as we think about the relationship between public and private provision of health care coverage. The three models:

- The Beveridge model is where the government owns and operates most medical facilities and health care costs are covered via taxes (e.g., New Zealand, Spain, and the United Kingdom).
- The Bismarck model is where the populace accesses health care via private facilities but must purchase health insurance, typically paid for through payroll deductions or taxes. The government then serves to

---

[13] Independent Healthcare Providers Network, "NHS Challenges Driving Demand."

regulate health insurance and mandate coverage for certain benefits (e.g., France, Germany, and Japan).
- The National Health Insurance model is where the private-sector entities provide care, but the government pays the bill with perhaps a small copay or deductible from the patient (e.g., Canada, Norway, and South Korea).

There are more than 185 countries in the world. Or in other words, there are more than 185 social science laboratories testing various versions of health care delivery, from fully comprehensive to surprisingly minimalist. The Legatum Institute prepared a comprehensive list of the best health care systems in the world, with the key measurements being "whether the populace is healthy and has access to services needed for maintaining good outcomes regarding illness, morbidity, and mortality."[14] The top ten, in order, were: Singapore, Japan, South Korea, Taiwan, China, Israel, Norway, Iceland, Sweden, and Switzerland. These are all worthwhile comparison points for the United States.

One should start with the presumption that the United States is and will remain a mixed system. It will be a complex hybrid of public-, private-, and NGO-sector institutions and resources. The public and private sectors are already intimately intertwined when it comes to providing health services. Private companies receive extensive revenue from governments, and they are subjected to extensive laws and regulations. In turn, for example, public-sector health facilities rely on the private sector for key items such as computer software, equipment, and pharmaceutical drugs.

Medicare and **Medicaid** are the primary governmental health insurance programs in the United States, and they cover about 40 percent of Americans.[15] There is a trend for public insurance programs to have a more private component. In the case of Medicaid, contracting with private plans can increase budget predictability for states. Almost 50 percent of Medicare beneficiaries are enrolled in **Medicare Advantage** plans run by private insurers, representing a doubling from just a decade ago, and over 70 percent of Medicaid beneficiaries are enrolled in a managed care plan operated by insurance companies.[16] Medicare and Medicaid are a significant source of profit for private insurers. Given the stagnancy of employer-sponsored insurance, public programs like Medicare and

---

[14] Legatum Institute, "Legatum Prosperity Index 2023."
[15] Centers for Medicare and Medicaid Services, *Access to Health Coverage*.
[16] Levitt, "Privatized Public Health Insurance."

Medicaid are now the major source of market growth for many private insurers.[17]

The private insurance industry now has a considerably larger financial stake in policy debates (e.g., level of government payments to Medicare Advantage plans) regarding public health insurance programs. As an example of potentially perverse incentives, Medicare Advantage plans, which are run by private insurers, have a financial incentive to identify more diagnoses for enrollees (called coding intensity) in order to raise risk-adjusted payments. Enrollment in such Medicare Advantage plans has grown substantially, and the number of extra benefits has increased. Beneficiaries in private Medicare Advantage plans can obtain extra benefits, typically without an added premium.

Many employers offer private health insurance coverage to their employees as a supplemental benefit. Providing high-quality private health care is typically a robust recruiting tool for employers as it helps attract the best candidates and can distinguish the businesses in a competitive hiring market. Employers use private-sector health care to stand out from competitors, increase employee morale, and improve talent retention. Private health insurance can be used to lower the cost of coinsurance, copays, deductibles, or specific treatments. There are also tax benefits for employers and employees. In the United States, employer costs for health insurance to cover employees or their dependents are 100 percent tax-deductible on corporate returns. Employees can also gain tax benefits by contributing to their health care costs using pretax money, which lowers the final tax bill for individual returns.

4.5   Across the Pond: The Complexity of US Health Care

From the patient perspective, the US health care system is extremely complex. Understanding the mix of public and private options can be confusing and time-consuming. Choosing individual/family insurance coverage can be a difficult decision, including factors such as financial capacity, health needs, and personal preferences. The process can be stressful. The distinct types of coverage include employer-based, private insurance, and government plans such as Medicare and Medicaid. Plans and prices can vary substantially depending on the insurer's policies and the policyholder's demographics. There are different rules for eligibility, funding, coverage, networks, enrollment dates, and out-of-pocket

---

[17] Freed et al., "Medicare Advantage in 2024."

responsibilities. There are also varying levels of coinsurance, copays, and deductibles. The contrasting types of coverage include fee-for-service systems, high-deductible plans, low- (or even practically zero) deductible plans, and managed care plans.

Adding to the complexity, if the public health care system is substandard or omits basic services, then the government or employers can offer access to supplemental health care insurance to fill in the gaps with private insurers in the open marketplace. Trained patient navigators can help people compare health insurance plans, assist with application processes, and provide on-demand answers. Navigators are either neutral, unbiased, or advocates of the patient; the key is they should not be biased toward or advocates of any health plans or providers.

From the provider perspective, there are byzantine sets of law, processes, and regulation regarding billing, coding, reimbursement, and usage. All of this drives administrative costs that are essentially additional overhead on top of the basic overhead. As noted in the previous chapter, as a percentage and in absolute terms, the United States spends far more on administrative costs than any other nation in the world, and these overhead costs are a key contributor.

The United States has relatively high private-sector health care costs. Part of this cost is driven by higher utilization, but as noted previously, the greater part of it is driven by higher cost per unit. Rather than the sheer number of procedures and tests in the United States, it is the average price per unit that makes health care so expensive, both in the public and private sectors. The private-sector costs are higher because of several nonvalue cost drivers detailed as follows:

Given the complexity of the system and the absence of any set prices for health services, providers have substantial leeway to charge whatever the demand will allow. As a result, the amount paid for an essentially identical medical service can vary significantly depending on the provider, the payer, the geographic region, and the type of coverage (e.g., private insurance, government programs, Medicaid, or Medicare). For example, Americans have a total cost per person for pharmaceutical drugs that is more than double the costs found in other advanced industrialized countries. While this is not the primary driver of health care costs, it is a striking area of overspending when compared to Canada and Europe, where drug prices are much more government-regulated. Also, because the United States is such a litigious society, including in the medical arena, malpractice insurance tends to be relatively expensive for private-sector entities, and health care professionals often have to practice "defensive" medicine, which can be especially inefficient and unnecessarily risk averse.

4.6 The Role of Government with Private-Sector Providers

The concept of health system stewardship means that governments should take responsibility for protecting the public interest in health care and have situational awareness of what is happening in the private sector. The governmental entity must develop a robust capacity to assess the strategic needs of the investments and contracted services, the cost efficiency and value for expenditures, and the long-term fiscal stability. Engaging the private sector in the provision of a public good like societal health naturally raises questions related to accountability, capacity, efficiency, governance, quality, and responsibility. With regard to the private health sector, the onus is still on governments to provide guidance, regulation, and accountability. Private health providers require performance monitoring as, inevitably, some providers are underqualified and will perform poorly.

Investment and capacity building are needed in developing effective evaluation criteria, contract management monitoring, and enforcement systems. Tools for government to measure and increase quality in the private sector include accreditation, credentialing, licensure, and regulation. Contracts with private-sector providers should clearly define metrics, measurements, price points, and the scope of the services. It should also be clear how contractors are selected and evaluated; integrity in procurement is essential. Government entities dispensing substantial amounts of money have to safeguard their integrity. Transparency, oversight, and accountability are crucial to proper governance of private-sector contracts. This generates increased public trust. To avoid even the perception of corruption in public procurement, it is essential to award contracts in a clear, open, and transparent manner.

If it is using private-sector providers, then the government has to ensure that health disparities remain an area of focus. Health equity is a complex issue requiring multiple stakeholders to effectively address. Traditional efforts have generally featured governments (e.g., county and state public health agencies). There are a large number of social programs available for enrollment including Children's Health Insurance Program, Supplemental Nutrition Assistance Program, Temporary Assistance for Needy Families, and Women, Infants, and Children. However, the private sector can play a significant role in advancing health equity.

In terms of its mandate and mission, the private sector is typically not set up to support public health goals. Moreover, the private sector tends to treat healthier, better-resourced patients relative to the government. Government has to ensure that collaborators from the private health sector are attuned to equity concerns. For any PPP, building community-level capability is crucial to creating, scaling, and sustaining a public health initiative. Addressing health equities requires knowledge of the local population coupled with maintaining long-standing trusting relationships with the community/neighborhood. Providers should meet patients where they are (e.g., barber shops, churches, community centers, farmers' markets, and malls), and the feedback of community stakeholders should be sought and incorporated.

As part of the private sector and its equity efforts, there is a diverse collection of large socially oriented nonprofit organizations (e.g., donor-funded institutions and faith-based providers) focused on health care. Examples in the United States include the American Diabetes Association, American Heart Association, American Red Cross, the United Way, and thousands of churches of diverse sizes drawn from various denominations. NGOs can be cost-effective and high-performing, while delivering equitable care. Often, they are the most impactful in reaching into communities and positively impacting disadvantaged populations. The government can be more creative in contracting with NGOs to set up provision for health care services and setting specific targets for improvement.

One form of collaboration involves governments contracting for medical services with private-sector companies. In turn, there are two submodels: (i) contracting out, where contractors have full responsibility for delivery of services, and (ii) contracting in, where contractors only manage select subsets within a governmental entity. These approaches can help cut costs, tap into specialized experts, and increase efficiency, while still allowing the governmental entity to lead higher-level management and oversight. For example, in order to cut patient wait times, Britain's National Health Service is doing more private-sector outsourcing of routine eye, hip, and knee surgeries. In addition, health care privatization is the process of transferring the provision of public services to private-sector entities.

Disruptive innovation typically yields benefits for many parts of the US economy, but in health care, the results are mixed, so the central policy challenge becomes how to encourage value-adding innovation for patients, providers, and payers without the medical or fiscal downsides.[18] Effectively leveraging the innovative capabilities and strategic resources of the private sector is critical to successfully pursuing the digital transformation of the health care sector. In this regard, we have to distinguish between "good

---

[18] Cutler and Song, "Private Investment."

innovation" and "bad innovation." Sometimes innovators can destroy value more rapidly than they create it, so health care leaders should encourage beneficial client-facing innovation. The private sector usually pays higher salaries, allowing it to draw talented, innovative health workers from the public workforce, and these entities usually find it less challenging to integrate new innovations.

As another crucial avenue for the private sector to improve the overall health care ecosystem, many health care startups are funded via private equity and venture capital, which benefit from a set of favorable tax rules. There has been extensive private-sector investment in health care delivery organizations, particularly in terms of new primary care models (e.g., addressing social determinants, intensified patient outreach, utilizing more efficient care modalities and settings, better integration of technology).[19] Many private-sector innovation models target the Medicare population, but some also focus on Medicaid patients as well.

The private sector, especially the technology companies, can be used in growth areas such as artificial intelligence, digitalization, machine learning, and telehealth. In terms of innovation, collection and sharing of data (e.g., analytics, geospatial observations, and surveillance dashboards) is increasingly important in PPPs. A significant challenge, faced by traditional collaborative health care partnerships, is the lack of infrastructure to collect, organize, share, and analyze data. Data flows should be bidirectional and real-time between the public and private entities.

Chapter Summary

This chapter highlights the importance of integrating universal and privatized health care systems to enhance the quality, accessibility, and equity of care. By balancing the strengths of public and private sectors, health care systems can mitigate the challenges of long wait times and limited resources often associated with universal health care while leveraging the innovation and efficiency of privatized options. Public–private partnerships emerge as a pivotal strategy for addressing health disparities, improving resource allocation, and ensuring financial sustainability. These partnerships demonstrate potential for enhancing health care delivery, particularly in underserved areas, by combining public accountability with private-sector agility and expertise. The COVID-19 pandemic underscored the power of collaboration, highlighting how private entities can supplement public health

---

[19] Landon, Weinreb, and Bitton, "Primary Care Delivery."

efforts during crises. It offered a superb example of how PPPs can be used to provide health services, with implications for key governance challenges, operational success, and financial probability.

The chapter also underscores the importance of transparency, equitable risk-sharing, and mutual trust in building effective collaborations. By incorporating advanced technologies like artificial intelligence and data analytics, PPPs can further optimize health care outcomes. While challenges remain – such as ensuring alignment with public health goals and addressing equity concerns – the potential for mixed systems to deliver comprehensive, high-quality care is undeniable. Ultimately, a hybrid model that leverages the unique strengths of public and private health care systems offers a pragmatic path toward achieving universal health coverage and improving health equity on a global scale. This collaborative approach aligns innovation with inclusivity, paving the way for a more effective, efficient, and equitable health care future.

CHAPTER 5

Health Needs to Be about People, Not Politics

Insights

- Partisanship and polarization can negatively impact collective and individual health outcomes.
- It is important to not be biased or partisan when considering the role of partisanship in health care policy.
- There is a general consensus on the importance of value-based care models.
- The system would benefit from more personalized/precision medicine and less polarization in health care.
- Data and technology offer a pathway toward less partisanship and polarization.

In this chapter, we assess US health care politics and policy, explaining how health care became such an ideological/partisan issue. We also discuss the need to align solutions across party lines and to prioritize patients in health care solutions. The US health care system faces several challenges in achieving universal health coverage and better health outcomes. This includes political ideologies that prioritize argumentation over solutions, resistance to resources shifting in order to achieve broader health coverage, and a diverse socioeconomic landscape, all of which can make it complicated to come to a consensus on health care policies. Additionally, the significant role of employer-based plans and private insurance creates a complex, hybrid system that often leaves many confused. Not surprisingly, confusion and uncertainty are enablers of polarization.

Hyper-partisanship exacerbates these challenges by framing health care as an ideological issue rather than a public good, leading to mistrust in public health initiatives and hindering collaborative policymaking. As a consequence, partisan divides can negatively influence health behaviors, generate self-imposed limitations on access to services, and impair overall public health outcomes. Efforts to foster bipartisan health care policies could include establishing clear, shared goals, focusing on priority health issues, engaging stakeholders across the political spectrum, and promoting accountability, responsibility, and transparency in policymaking. Community engagement and collaboration among health care providers, insurers, and policy makers are essential to addressing the needs of diverse populations effectively. As discussed, data and technology offer additional robust pathways out of the morass of polarization.

A highly partisan, polarized United States is not good for the health of the country's politics, policy, or health care. Fortunately, there are policy techniques and technology tools that strengthen our capacity to make people happier and healthier by being less partisan and polarized. The big three health care programs in the United States (Affordable Care Act [ACA], Medicaid, and Medicare) all suffer from excessive politicization.

5.1 Across the Pond: The Basis for Polarization

The UN has Sustainable Development Goals related to nations achieving universal health coverage. Almost all high-income countries have already reached the goals regarding health care, but the United States is a notable exception.[1] Among thirty-seven nations that are members of the Organisation for Economic Co-operation and Development (OECD), the United States is the only one that does not provide universal health care, either by constitutional right or in practice. Over the past eighty years, the United States has signed at least six international declarations and treaties recognizing a right to health care in some form. Two treaties were signed, ratified, and are legally binding under international law; two other treaties were signed but were never ratified; and two declarations were signed but are not legally binding.

There are philosophical and political challenges to moving the United States toward a universal health care coverage (UHC) system. Few countries in the world are as culturally complex, as ethnically/racially diverse, with such firmly held political/religious beliefs that can be quite different, and with a geographical area as large as the United States, which has a populace that spans the full range of the vast socioeconomic spectrum. Another part of the reason that the US health care system is so globally anomalous is the strong individualistic, capitalistic culture. Many in the United States are used to getting the care they want, when they want it, and

---

[1] Eozenou, Neelsen, and Pirlea, "Universal Health Coverage."

from whoever they want. This assumption is deeply ingrained in the culture. There is concern that having too strong of a government role in health care could stagnate entrepreneurship and innovation.

In the United States, it is unlikely that a full universal health care option could be funded solely by increasing taxes on the wealthy, so the financial burden on the middle class and working class would likely increase, either directly (i.e., income tax) or indirectly (e.g., via taxes on consumption or employers), which has serious political implications. Political leaders are usually reluctant to increase financial burdens directly and visibly on large voting blocks. Moreover, moving toward a UHC system could actually introduce more politics into health care as federal and state elected officials would generally have an even larger role in budgets, care decisions, expenses, regulations, and rules.

Given the lack of UHC, the result is a complex, hybrid system in the United States. It forces health care to be flexible and skilled enough to participate in multiple payment models, and it forces the US health care system to rely heavily on the private sector and employer insurance. Having insurance through one's employer is good until one loses it. A job loss is a triple negative impact, which causes: (i) loss of income, (ii) loss of health care, and (iii) lowered self-esteem. So, for all of its advantages, patient dependence on employer insurance has significant downsides. In contrast, the **Veterans Affairs Health System (VA)**, operated by the US Department of Veterans Affairs, serves former military members, and is an example of a government-run, single-payer health care provider. However, the VA system is costly and has uneven results. There seem to be no easy fixes that are fully effective.

The US Congressional Budget Office projects that federal government spending on health insurance will grow from the current 7 percent of gross domestic product (GDP) to a whopping 8.3 percent of GDP by 2033, which is a significant increase, especially when the goal is to reduce health expenditures.[2] A considerable proportion of US health expenditures are not tied to patient outcomes or even treatment per se. Instead, according to a McKinsey & Company report, about 25 percent of it goes to administrative functions.[3] Over the past fifty years, nearly every industry in the United States has achieved substantial gains in productivity – except the health care sector. Medical costs are projected to continue growing, which will impact governments and individuals. As noted, medical debt

---

[2] Congressional Budget Office, *Federal Subsidies for Health Insurance*.
[3] Sahni et al., "Administrative Simplification."

continues to be the top driver of personal bankruptcy in the United States. Furthermore, the relatively high cost and unevenness of health care fuel politicization.

Politics is not necessarily a prologue for partisanship, but the foundation for greater polarization has been present for some time. The sheer diversity of the United States, coupled with the continued challenges regarding access and affordability of the health care system, makes health policy a ripe venue for polarization. Polarization is often understood to be occurring when political parties move further and further apart on their ideological orientations, political views, and policy preferences. It also occurs when the collective electorate's views about parties, politics, and policies come to take on a bimodal distribution rather than the normal distribution. Those who are polarized come to love their partisan in-group and loathe the partisan out-group. Hyper-partisanship can undercut collective action because those with the most polarized identities are usually reluctant to accept incongruent information. The lack of moderates in the middle makes compromise, consensus, lawmaking, and policymaking considerably more challenging.

In conditions of polarization, beliefs and interests of society become concentrated at opposing extremes rather than along a steady continuum. Some distinguish polarization as being a collective phenomenon and partisanship as applying to the individual level, but for our purposes, they are essentially synonyms. "Extremification" involves the movement of attitudes and opinions regarding health care away from the center and toward more ideological extremes so that issues become "all or nothing."[4] This results in a hardening of positions, making effective consensus considerably more difficult to achieve. Partisanship has a corrosive effect upon levels of institutional trust and mutual respect, as well as the overall quality of public discourse.

5.2 Increasing Partisanship and Polarization

Over the past forty years, partisanship has increased in the United States. One study found that, from 1980 through 2008, survey respondents were more likely to say they "loved" their own party rather than "hated" the opposite party. By 2020, respondents were much more likely to say they "hated" the opposite party rather than "loved" their own party.[5] Moreover,

---

[4] Van Bavel et al., "Political Polarization and Health."
[5] Van Bavel et al., "Political Polarization and Health."

5.2 Increasing Partisanship and Polarization

in the United States, the "loathing" has become an even stronger factor than the "loving."[6] Partisanship and polarization are defining features of current US politics and policy,[7] and there is a trend toward affiliation-based decision-making.

Overall, the United States is currently in a negative feedback loop, with our elected officials amplifying the polarization. Increasingly, politics is seen as a type of warfare, with elections being viewed as a struggle between forces of good and forces of evil. Members of the other party are seen as enemies rather than as opponents. As one vivid example of these dynamics, a research study showed that a conservative physician in a predominantly liberal region had twice the likelihood of relocating than did their liberal counterpart; the reverse is also true for a liberal physician living in a conservative region.[8] At one level, this is not surprising and just represents the enduring human tendency of homophily (i.e., seeking out and associating with others who are similar). Yet, at another level, it shows that even physicians increasingly prefer to sort themselves geographically in ways that achieve greater philosophical and political alignment with the communities and patients they serve.

Health Care, essentially, has now become inherently political. The increasingly oppositional coalitions, constituencies, and lobbyists continue to impact health policy. Cycles of excessive partisanship undermine health care policy, and there is the danger of getting into a negative feedback loop where the existing levels of polarization drive even more polarization. While we may treat politics as a sport, health care is inherently different and should not be treated in the same way. For the past several decades, states have expanded their independence from the federal government regarding welfare programs, including those directly affecting health care (e.g., Medicaid). Health spending accounts for 25–35 percent of most state budgets.[9] That is a significant percentage. Moreover, there has been a growth in "partisan federalism," where states led by one party challenge the policies of the federal presidential administration from the other party.[10]

There is a distinction between politics and partisanship. At some fundamental level, health care has to involve politics because it inherently involves public policy and the allocation of resources. It is unrealistic to aim for an environment where health care policy is devoid of politics. For

---

[6] Finkel et al., "Political Sectarianism in America."
[7] Oberlander, "Polarization, Partisanship, and Health."
[8] Bonica et al., "Ideological Sorting of Physicians."   [9] Katz Olson, "Healthcare."
[10] Bulman-Pozen, "Partisan Federalism."

example, one inherent feature of health insurance is a practice of risk pooling where the healthy end up overpaying in order to help the unhealthy, allowing the former to ensure their own lower costs if they become sick in the future. The challenge is that short-term losers (i.e., those paying now) may object to this resource and wealth transfer to the short-term winners (i.e., those benefiting now), which makes these sorts of trade-offs politically difficult. Yet, the inherent presence of politics does not necessarily mean that there has to be partisanship and polarization regarding these decisions.

The potential for partisanship in health care is also higher because the subject areas are often so incredibly complex. Medical science is generally not characterized by absolutes, so there is an inherent degree of uncertainty in every fact and truth. This makes it relatively easy to argue for more extreme positions regarding health policy and medical science. In fact, polarization in this regard is not entirely new, but it has been amplified in the era of social media. We can convey public health information through traditional, curated channels, but there are now thousands of alternative media sources. "Motivated reasoning" occurs when the public interprets media information about a given health law or policy in divergent ways that correspond to their different partisan identities.[11] The democratization and diversification of media sources lends itself to the growing trend of motivated reasoning that allows partisans to interpret health care laws, policies, regulation, and science in ways that fit their own polarized views.

Figure 5.1 captures these basic dynamics. Due to its tremendous complexity (public, private, and NGO actors at the local, state, and federal levels), consequentiality (e.g., literally life and death issues), and size (approximately $4 trillion), the US health care system generates substantial challenges and opportunities. This requires that public-sector leaders, with input from an enormous variety of individual and organizational voices, make large resource-allocation decisions. It is natural and not necessarily unhealthy that politics comes into the process. The trouble for society and for productive public discourse occurs when politics devolves into partisanship (including becoming hyper-partisan) and that further devolves into polarization (including becoming hyperpolarized). The final unfortunate landing spot is "extremification." Fortunately, at least before the disagreements reach the most extreme stage, there are ways to end the vicious downward spiral and create, instead, an upward spiral. As we discuss, one pathway is through greater use of data, analytics, machine

---

[11] Jacobs, Mettler, and Zhu, "Pathways of Policy Feedback."

5.2 Increasing Partisanship and Polarization

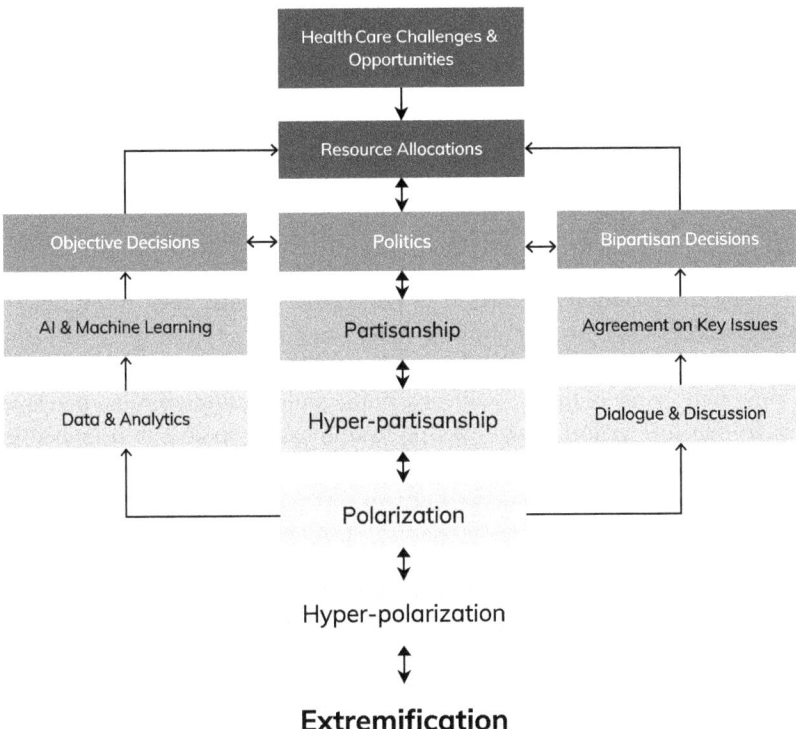

Figure 5.1 Pathway to and from polarization in US health care policymaking

learning, and artificial intelligence to make more evidence-based, fact-driven, and objective decisions. Another positive pathway is to have more open dialogue to reach agreement on key issues (e.g., health care coverage for the working class, increasing internet connectivity, which is crucial for telemedicine, and reducing opioid addiction). This can lead to more bipartisan decision-making, laws, and regulations. The double-arrowed lines in the diagram capture the typically fluid and reciprocal (rather than unidirectional) nature of US politics.

Trusted voices are essential to addressing the concerns of some parts of the population; polarization has a corrosive effect, in that it eats away at the quantity and impact of those who are trusted. Health Care professionals (e.g., dentists, nurses, pharmacists, and physicians) have historically been among the most trusted sources of health information for Americans. Health agencies also engage actively, directly, and publicly with trusted voices from the community. However, the number of these voices is diminishing, and those who remain have diminished influence. Why? Because political polarization often determines who people trust and listen to, as well as how they interpret risk. Elevated levels of distrust lead to deadweight loss (i.e., it imposes a societal cost without any societal benefit). Distrust, in the form of this deadweight loss, essentially imposes a massive "tax" on our health care system, making communication of accurate, important health care information considerably more costly and time-consuming, while ultimately, it is also less effective.

If the conversation stops short of rabid partisanship, then having arguments and discussions of politics in health care can be healthy. In fact, the best policies often emerge in the wake of robust dialogue and discussion. Conversely, some of the most adverse public policies often result when laws or regulations reflect only one philosophical or political perspective. Human beings are not all angels and saints, and recognizing that government is composed of and run by humans, there is no reason to assume that federal, state, or local governmental units possess an infallibility that places them above reproach. Governments often yield – or are on the cusp of yielding – awful laws and policies in health care. Normal, healthy levels of partisanship and politics can help elevate the quality of existing health care policies or prevent the adoption of adverse ones. Unfortunately, these debates tend to be characterized by extremification and hyper-partisanship.

5.3 Polarization Hurts Patient Health and Policymaking

Partisanship can shape health behaviors and even health outcomes. As noted, political polarization can impact who individuals trust, how they assess health risks, and, ultimately, what health care products/services they access. Accordingly, it is reasonable to question whether America's growing political polarization could be exacerbating its health outcomes gap, relative to other nations. As individuals move to more partisan political positions, there can be a decline in individual and public health, including lower participation in healthy behaviors and preventive practices.[12] If community norms are misinformed or unhealthy, members are more likely

---

[12] Finkel et al., "Political Sectarianism in America."

5.3 Polarization's Impact on Health and Policy

to engage in unhealthy behavior. At the most basic level, hyper-partisanship and polarization can make people feel mentally unwell by increasing feelings of isolation and stress. The feeling of being in an adversarial relationship with and politically distant from fellow citizens and neighbors heightens the risk of depression and anxiety disorders.

Consider this tangible example. Longitudinal data analysis reveals that in the time since Democrats passed the Patient Protection and Affordable Care Act, Republicans were considerably less likely than Democrats to enroll in the program.[13] From the very beginning of the law's enactment, Republicans have been less likely than Democrats or Independents to join the ACA's insurance exchanges.[14] Thus, partisanship is driving different health behaviors. As another vivid example, COVID-19 ultimately became a partisan pandemic. The pandemic is essentially a master class in observing the risks to health policy that are associated with polarization.

Research on the determinants of health should consider incorporating the role of polarization. Much like the social determinants of health (SDOH), political polarization is a macro-level factor that can aggravate public health risks at the collective and individual levels. We could call this the cultural/political determinants of health. The political determinants of health focus on how policies, politics, and procedures guide population health practices within a community. Political polarization can essentially serve as a national-level "preexisting condition" for the US health care ecosystem. It is important to understand and mitigate the potential health risks attendant to global political polarization, and just as with SDOH, policy leaders should aim to mitigate the potentially harmful effects of polarization on health. Removing the hyper-partisan influence on health care would be like lancing a cancerous tumor.

Partisanship and polarization are now consistent features of the US health policy landscape. Since political debates on health care laws are increasingly fought along partisan lines, political polarization risks obstructing the implementation of legislation designed to keep Americans healthy. Hyper-partisanship can cause conflicts regarding health care issues to spread in scale and scope. These polarized disputes can reshape a law's post-enactment trajectory of implementation and interpretation, leading to prolonged fights over new laws that persist long after their enactment, creating post-enactment trajectories and making it considerably more challenging to encourage adoption and build

---

[13] Lerman, Sadin, and Trachtman, "Policy Uptake as Political Behavior."
[14] Trachtman, "Polarization, Participation, and Premiums."

popularity. Partisanship can expand the scope of conflict on health care policy to a broader and deeper set of institutions and issues. Polarization can also generate partisan conflict in health care issues that previously had been bipartisan or apolitical. It also seems to widen differences in state health law and policies.

Given this state of affairs, what can be done? Is it feasible to move US health care policies and policymaking to a less partisan, less polarized state? How can we build trust in the health care system, including acknowledging the concerns of others and achieving consensus on at least some policies?

5.4 Reducing Polarization – Generally

As with almost any policy legislation, some people may be better off from a given health care law, and others may be worse off. Ultimately, when it comes to health care, rather than thinking about political philosophy, most Americans are more focused on their own specific benefits (e.g., coverage, deductibles, quality). People typically ask how any given policy will impact them and/or their family. Because of these highly consequential resource allocation decisions (e.g., health care coverage is sometimes literally a life-or-death issue, or it can be the difference between bankruptcy and avoiding financial ruin), there are profound challenges for any attempts, no matter how earnest those attempts might be, to depolarize health care. These include difficulty achieving consensus on optimal evidence-based practices, opposition from hyper-partisan forces, resistance from entrenched industry players that benefit from the status quo, loss of funding from good programs that rely on political support, and the conundrum of ensuring accountability without strong political accountability/oversight.

Ideally, there should be more personalization and less polarization in health care. Patient-centered policies and personalized medicine should be prioritized over party ideologies. Can partisan divides be bridged? We want to encourage two versions of ourselves: (i) the self-interested consumer (i.e., seeking to gain the best possible family and individual benefit for health dollars spent) and (ii) the altruistic society member (i.e., seeking to make sure fellow members of the country and community are realizing value in health care). We ideally want to discourage the extremely partisan version of ourselves, as this includes a tendency to elevate doctrine over value. As part of this, there should be a culture of collaboration among patients, providers, payers, pharmaceuticals, pharmacies, and policy makers, with a primary focus on effective care delivery.

5.4 Reducing Polarization – Generally

To restore, build, and maintain trust in public health institutions and officials, it is important to have greater accountability, responsibility, and transparency. To rebuild trust among citizens, we should encourage openness regarding policymaking and implementation. It is important to be candid about the uncertainties regarding medicine, and research and development; scientific knowledge is fallible. We should consistently implement evidence-based guidelines for care that prioritize patient outcomes, while promoting transparency in health care funding, decision-making, and management.

The public favorability of a policy often depends on how the media frames legislation. We should do more to frame the situation positively by focusing on those who are following personal health and public health guidelines rather than focusing on those who are failing to do so. We can utilize admired and respected civil and social leaders as trusted voices who are above – or at least adjacent to – partisanship and politics. Community, entertainment, military, religious, and sports leaders can help promote health messages and positive compliance norms. The potential benefits of depolarizing health care include elevating public trust in the health care system, focusing on long-term health strategies instead of short-term political gains, improving patient outcomes via evidence-based practices, and increasing efficiency in care delivery by minimizing bureaucratic hurdles.

Especially at the local and state levels, there should be increased public engagement via community forums and workshops educating people on health care issues. It is important to build coalitions across party lines. Specific approaches include (i) establishment of bipartisan health care committees to encourage dialogue among different partisan perspectives and political parties and (ii) creation of independent health policy boards that are at least somewhat insulated from day-to-day political influence. To address local needs effectively, as was often done during the COVID-19 crisis, there should be partnerships between health care providers, payers, and policy makers. It is important for key stakeholders to be engaged in the depoliticization process, including the use of community forums, peer groups, and listening sessions.

Mental health is one potential area of consensus. There is rising demand for psychiatric services among adults and children, which is driving growth in behavioral health urgent care clinics across the United States. Nearly 25 percent of the US population utilizes some form of behavioral health services.[15] About 8 percent of visitors to emergency departments are seeking mental health support,[16] so funneling some of these patients to urgent care clinics can relieve pressure on emergency rooms. Walk-in mental health clinics offer a new crisis center model (e.g., a shift of mental health care to urgent care spaces) that can address critical gaps and improve patient outcomes. Remote counseling and therapy sessions continue to grow in prevalence, providing increased mental health care via telehealth services and virtual care.

Opioid abuse prevention is another potential area of consensus. In the United States, an incredible 81,000 annual overdose deaths are linked to opioids.[17] The continued epidemic of opioid abuse disorders stimulates greater use of non-opioid therapies and the reshaping of pain management. The alternative therapies involve a wave of non-opioid drugs (e.g., ketamine, psilocybin) and non-pharmacological interventions that can deliver effective pain relief without the addiction and overdose risks associated with opioids. Because of the ubiquity of the problem, population health policies are being developed and implemented at federal, state, local, community, neighborhood, and organizational levels. Opioid addiction prevention is an area that is ripe for data-driven, depolarized decision-making, offering an exemplar for other health policies.

5.5 Reducing Polarization – Specific Examples

The idea of reducing polarization seems excellent in theory, but is there any chance it would work in practice, particularly given the current hyper-partisan environment? Or would it be like a quest to find a mermaid, minotaur, or unicorn? Fortunately, there are specific, tangible cases of highly successful bipartisan health care policy development, adoption, and implementation. It starts with shared objectives. Examples of bipartisan goals in health care include: (i) addressing mental health disorders, (ii) improving health care infrastructure in rural areas, (iii) increasing access to affordable health coverage for working-class, uninsured populations, (iv) providing noncriminal treatment options to those with substance use disorders, and (v) reducing prescription drug prices via increased competition and transparency.

Even with the ACA, states from across a diverse political spectrum have opted to expand Medicaid, demonstrating widespread agreement on the

---

[15] Jain, "2023 Trends," 50. [16] Villas-Boas et al., "Emergency Department Visits."
[17] National Institute on Drug Abuse, *Drug Overdose Deaths*.

5.5 Reducing Polarization – Specific Examples

value of health access. Arkansas and Indiana, two states that are considered relatively conservative politically, have successfully implemented Medicaid expansion with strong bipartisan support, increasing coverage and improving outcomes. Hopefully, state governments will continue to develop affordable care by encouraging smart Medicaid expansion or targeted subsidies for low-income individuals, especially the "working poor."

Here are other examples of bipartisan legislation and policymaking, as well as specific issues where there seems to be broad agreement that spans much of the partisan spectrum in the United States:

- The Children's Health Insurance Program has generally garnered bipartisan support; it provides health coverage to children in families with incomes that are too low to afford relatively expensive private coverage but too high to be eligible for Medicaid.
- The 21st Century Cures Act was designed to accelerate medical product development, bringing new innovations (e.g., devices and drugs) to patients more quickly; it was drafted and adopted with overwhelming support from both major parties.
- The Opioid Crisis Response Act addressed the opioid epidemic with smart measures including prevention and treatment strategies; it was implemented with strong bipartisan agreement. Integrating treatment for mental health and substance use disorder into primary care is an idea that can garner widespread political support.
- The Mental Health Parity and Addiction Equity Act mandated that insurance plans treat mental health services equal to physical health services.
- Due in large part to public demand for lower drug costs, the Affordable Drug Pricing Act implemented bipartisan pricing reforms on pharmaceuticals. It promotes a reduction in prescription drug prices by allowing the importation of drugs from other countries and encouraging price negotiation.
- There is often broad agreement on creating and supporting community health center initiatives, perhaps because they are such locally oriented resources. The Community Health Center Fund has bipartisan support, providing essential funding for health services in underserved areas. Community health workers are widely recognized as valuable for bridging gaps in health care access by providing education, information, and support to vulnerable populations directly in their communities and neighborhoods.

- There is bipartisan support for decentralized decision-making, empowering local communities to make health care decisions particular to their own needs and reducing reliance on federal guidance.
- There is bipartisan support for transparent pricing models, creating standardized and clear pricing for medical procedures and services, thereby enabling patients to make considerably more informed choices.
- There is bipartisan support for the value of urgent care clinics. There are currently over 14,000 urgent care centers in the United States, with a growth rate of 7 percent for new centers.[18] Urgent care facilities help manage common health issues and those needing immediate care for injuries. They help prevent approximately 25 million emergency room visits annually, reducing the burden on emergency rooms, while saving patients money and time.[19]
- Telehealth often provides increased access, convenience, cost-effectiveness, patient engagement, and tracking. For example, it avoids the time, expense, and logistical inconvenience of travel. There is broad political support for increased communications infrastructure to support virtual health, and telemedicine is politically popular.
- Health data interoperability allows effective and efficient sharing of patient health records and additional medical data across providers, which improves care coordination and reduces administrative burdens. The lack of interoperability imposes a deadweight loss on the system, so there is consensus to increase the ability to share and aggregate data and other information.
- There is a general consensus on the importance of **value-based care** models, incentivizing providers to shift from volume-based (i.e., **fee-for-service**) models to a focus on patient outcomes and quality.

Of course, this kind of broad agreement does not happen by accident, and it is not self-generating. It takes significant effort. There are several keys to developing and adopting bipartisan health care legislation:

- Clearly defined goals to address pressing health issues impacting a broad constituency.
- Diligent stakeholder engagement, seeking and incorporating feedback from patients, providers, payers, and advocacy groups.
- Data-driven decision-making, relying on analytics, evidence, and research to support any proposed measures.

---

[18] Urgent Care Association, "Nature of Urgent Care," 3.
[19] Urgent Care Association, "Nature of Urgent Care."

- Focus on cost-effectiveness and long-term financial viability to ensure that the policies can be maintained over time.

Patient centricity should be the guiding light and lodestar for creating, maintaining, and growing the quality and quantity of bipartisan policy-making. Policies should begin and end with the patient in mind. As part of this, we need to substantially educate patients. More knowledgeable patients are likely to be less polarized patients. Patients will increasingly take charge of their own health decisions as greater access to consumer data (e.g., clinical data, claims data, consumer demographics, and SDOH) facilitates consumer-centric health care.

Patient demand and the need for digital health care tools (e.g., patient portals, self-service features) is robust. Increasing patients' access to digital engagement tools will benefit both patients and providers. As one form of patient empowerment, consumers will increasingly be able to purchase drugs directly from manufacturers. Drug companies are pioneering the use of direct-to-consumer strategies, beginning at the front of drug life cycles rather than just the backend, when patent exclusivity expires. The principal challenge to consumer education remains the astounding complexity of the US health care system. For example, not only are many Americans uninsured or underinsured, but many are unsure of their exact coverage levels and how to utilize their benefits. Thus, continued education and learning is needed so that patients become better-informed consumers of health-related policy and politics, which will ultimately yield benefits including less partisanship and reduced polarization.

5.6 Data and Technology as Enablers of Depolarization

Greater utilization of data and technology offers a pathway to better medicine and less partisanship. In this regard, there are many exciting developments in health care and medicine. The explosive volume of health data is fueling rapid medical and scientific advances. To establish wellness plans that drive long-lasting improvements and meet quality program requirements, providers will need a more comprehensive, holistic view of patient data and overall health. Algorithms exist now that can help clinicians predict and prevent adverse patient events, drawing upon thousands of similar cases to create actionable alerts, personalized recommendations, and smart rules.

Data can improve clinical decision-making, validate treatment decisions, and inform reimbursement decisions. Both the quantity and quality of data are critical. And based on this data, there will be a continued shift to predictive measures to cope with aging demographics, booming populations, and uncertain economies. We can use predictive analytics to achieve a better understanding of cost drivers. Personalized health care aims to move the patient's health from reactive to preventative, and precision medicine will require leveraging the power of AI, analytics, and data (e.g., tailored communication strategies and wellness plans).

As noted, **data interoperability** references the ability of different systems and technologies to share and process information effectively. Standardization refers to the use of consistent formats and protocols when exchanging and managing data. Interoperability and standardization have become increasingly important as health systems exhibit greater utilization of digital solutions, making it essential to seamlessly exchange and interpret data. The **Internet of Medical Things (IoMT)** refers to a network of interconnected applications, devices, platforms, and software to collect, store, analyze, and exchange health data. Data interoperability, standardization, and the IoMT all point toward the potential for a more fact-driven, depoliticized way of making health policy.

Data can strengthen value-based payment models, helping to control abuse, fraud, and waste. The ironic downside is that growth in data also means growth in the potential for misuse, neglect, and theft. Connected health systems, telemedicine, and wearable devices have introduced new vulnerabilities, and given the high valuation of patient data on illicit markets, bad actors are more motivated than ever to penetrate security systems. The Internet of Things has significantly broadened the scale and scope of patient privacy concerns. Many experts note that the health care sector is an industry that suffers more heavily from the negative impact of data security violations, with the average breach costing over $10 million.[20] A focus on robust cybersecurity systems has become a top trend in health care. Thus, data growth is not a free lunch; it contains inherent dangers and downsides. However, the upside potential, including the prospect of more data-driven decision-making, exceeds the downside risks.

Severe resource constraints are often an essential fuel for polarization. Fortunately, technological innovations in health care are helping to ease these constraints by allowing the system to do more with less. The health care sector is experiencing a transformative surge of innovation, with cutting-edge technologies reshaping data utilization, medical processes, patient care, operational efficiency, and strategic investments. Much of

---

[20] World Economic Forum, "Cyberattacks."

this innovation is being funded by angel investors, family offices, investment banks, private equity, and venture capital. The future of health care technology will require creating a sustainable ecosystem where innovation, investment security, and human expertise operate in harmony.

As an example of easing resource constraints, provider organizations are developing new, innovative technologies that help combat physician burnout and the rising care costs. Automating repetitive tasks like billing, patient record management, and scheduling can improve overall record accuracy, reduce administrative bottlenecks, and streamline workflow. Virtual health care sessions are increasingly being delivered remotely by human therapists, and there is a growing use of chatbots to provide on-demand, instantaneous support.

Use of **remote patient monitoring (RPM)** is growing. Remote patient monitoring provides clinicians with real-time data for case management, and it has proven capable of reducing hospital readmissions, while freeing up hospital beds for those with greater needs. Through tools such as connected home health equipment, mobile apps, and wearable devices, RPM allows providers to continuously track patient metrics (e.g., medication adherence, vital signs) outside the clinical context. This information allows clinicians to make highly informed decisions relatively quickly, which can avoid serious complications and hospital admissions. The home is the new hospital; the home is the new hospital room. Hospital-at-home programs allow for high-level care, even outside the hospital setting.

The health care sector is increasingly embracing digital innovations such as augmented reality (AR) and virtual reality (VR) to transform care, education, and operations. Originally, AR and VR were primarily technologies for entertainment (e.g., gaming), but they are now powerful tools being leveraged for key tasks such as advanced patient treatment methods, noninvasive training simulations, and pain management.[21] By providing a controlled, immersive setting, VR can also assist patients in managing anxiety, depression, and other debilitating mental health conditions.

Personalized/precision medicine improves care while avoiding or at least reducing the trial-and-error process usually associated with treatments. Brain–computer interfaces offer the next generation of insertable and wearable health-tech devices for ailments such as chronic pain management, epilepsy, and paralysis. Genomics and gene editing are exciting frontiers in molecular-level care, enabling the use of targeted treatments for genetic conditions (e.g., cystic fibrosis, Huntington's disease, muscular

---

[21] Lier et al., "Effect Modifiers of Virtual Reality."

dystrophy). "Clustered regularly interspaced short palindromic repeats" is a breakthrough technology, which allows researchers and scientists to selectively modify the DNA of living organisms, and it is increasingly being used in the fight against cancer and cardiovascular disease. Minimally invasive procedures, which provide faster recovery, fewer complications, and reduced pain, will continue to replace traditional highly invasive surgeries.

We generally think of technology in an apolitical way. Yet, because they can ease resource constraints, technological innovations in health care offer a pathway to less polarization. For similar reasons, the same is true for data. We can then combine analytics, data, and technology to drive artificial intelligence and machine learning, which we will discuss in more detail in the next chapter. Working in unison, these tools can be depolarizing.

Chapter Summary

In summary, this chapter underscores the intricate and polarized landscape of the US health care system, which stands in stark contrast to the global movement toward universal health coverage. Despite signing international treaties recognizing a right to health care, the United States remains the only OECD nation lacking a UHC framework, primarily due to cultural, financial, and political challenges. The ingrained capitalistic and individualistic values prevalent in American society contribute to a complex health care model that is heavily reliant on employer-sponsored plans and private insurance. This chapter highlights how political polarization has exacerbated health care challenges, leading to entrenched partisan divides that hinder effective policymaking.

As health care becomes increasingly politicized, issues that should be approached collaboratively are instead framed as battlegrounds for ideological warfare. This polarization not only complicates the development of sound health care policy but also negatively impacts public trust and health outcomes, as individuals begin to make health decisions based on partisan affiliations rather than evidence-based practices. However, there are potential pathways to mitigate polarization through increased transparency, stakeholder engagement, and a rigorous focus on patient-centered policies. Prioritizing collaboration across party lines, while utilizing data and technological innovations, could pave the way for more effective health care policy and delivery. By fostering norms of accountability, partnership, and trust, the United States could move toward a more nonpartisan and efficient health care system, ultimately improving health outcomes for all citizens.

CHAPTER 6

The Affordable Care Act: Why Is It So Unaffordable?

Insights

- The pricing for medical care continues to lack transparency for both patients and employers, with similar products and services varying substantially for unclear reasons.
- Underuse is a more serious issue in US health care than overuse.
- Universal health care in the United States needs to be accompanied by cost containment because it would bankrupt the nation if the federal government simply insured everyone under the current system.
- Although some preventive services and disease management programs often save money, many times they do not.
- The basic political problem is that these cost savings in the US health care system are not free, so there is, almost invariably, at least some zero-sum element.

In this chapter, we take a careful look at the reasons why the Affordable Care Act (ACA), in its original form, failed to live up to its promises of reducing the key metric: *costs* of care. While it is impossible to know if the ACA would have reduced costs if it was allowed to roll out as planned, the focus in this chapter is on the here and now – to identify solutions for reviving the Act and moving toward more bipartisan health care policy. A key theme in this chapter is the value of ideas over ideology to encourage bipartisan solutions. As part of this, we examine the ACA's tumultuous journey as landmark legislation that sought to revolutionize and transform the US health care system. The Act's ambitious goals aimed to extend insurance coverage to millions of uninsured citizens while controlling and ideally reducing the rising costs of health care services. Early challenges faced during the ACA's implementation included a failed website launch, overly complex choices between insurance options, and the struggle to attract younger, healthier individuals into the insurance pool.

6 The Affordable Care Act: Why Is It So Unaffordable?

Despite a notable reduction in the uninsured population, the ACA's outcomes have fallen short of projections, revealing significant gaps in competition, cost-effectiveness, enrollment, and simplification. We analyze the two primary components of the ACA's coverage expansion (Medicaid and subsidized exchanges), while highlighting the complexities and unintended consequences of the ACA for governments, companies, and patients. The presence of externalities and misaligned incentives has been particularly problematic. We conclude by looking to the future and considering how the role of emerging technologies like artificial intelligence (AI) is reshaping health care delivery and addressing the ongoing challenges faced by the ACA. This chapter provides a critical reflection on the ACA's legacy, offering insights into both its achievements and the significant remaining obstacles in the quest for accessible, affordable, high-quality health care in the United States.

6.1 ACA Beginnings, Launch, Goals, and Achievements

The ACA aimed to make health care more affordable by providing insurance coverage for millions of uninsured Americans and by controlling costs for medical services. The ACA was primarily designed to help make health insurance affordable for the relatively small percentage of people who buy it from the individual market. In the pre-ACA period, insurance companies could consider an applicant's health status when making decisions about whether to provide coverage and what price to set for premiums. Insurance companies often denied coverage for those even with relatively minor current or prior health problems, or if they agreed to provide coverage, they often set premiums at a prohibitively expensive level. The ACA implemented two key requirements: guaranteed issue (i.e., insurance companies must sell insurance to anyone who applies) and community rating (i.e., people of the same age, who buy similar insurance, must pay similar prices). These two provisions made it feasible, for example, for an older person with cancer to be able to purchase insurance. The ACA initially required all Americans to purchase health insurance or face a penalty, but that provision was eventually eliminated.

At its launch, the ACA portal quickly became known as unreliable and not user-friendly, adding to the stress of shopping for health insurance. On the first day, only six people in the United States successfully chose health insurance plans and completed enrollment using the ACA website.[1] It took

---
[1] Dwyer, "Obamacare on First Day."

nearly two months before the ACA website became functional for enrollment, and over a decade later, glitches still remained, with people sometimes being enrolled or switched to different plans without their consent. Although the percentage of individuals without insurance has gone down, enrollment in the exchanges is considerably below projections. Back then, the Congressional Budget Office estimated that insurers selling plans in the exchanges, which are the ACA's primary health insurance hubs, would enroll 25 million people over the next decade. However, average enrollment has been stuck at only 10 million people since 2015, which is about 60 percent below expectations.

The ACA had two primary components of its coverage expansion: Medicaid and subsidized exchanges. Because the vast majority of the people who gained coverage via the ACA enrolled in Medicaid, some have referred to it as the "Medicaid Expansion Act."[2] Thus, much of the net reduction in the uninsured is attributable to Medicaid growth. Historically, Medicaid is a welfare benefits program that typically served individuals with disabilities, low-income children, pregnant women, and seniors. The expansion of Medicaid has the potential to crowd out services for the more vulnerable populations that the program has traditionally served.

The ACA did not have strong success in attracting healthy young people into the exchange insurance pools. Those younger covered lives are crucially needed to offset the cost of older, sicker enrollees. The enrollees on the exchange are far older and poorer than anticipated. It is important to guard against the ACA's individual market transforming into a highly subsidized source of coverage for older and sicker patients. A death spiral occurs when a health plan takes on more and more sick patients, while losing more and more healthy patients. Due to the inherent trade-offs needed (e.g., young vs. old, healthy vs. sick, wealthy vs. poor), it is incredibly hard to change the US health care system in ways that both broaden coverage and generate substantial savings. The problem is that potential savings in the US health care system are not free; they often come along with cost cuts or coverage decisions that would be extremely expensive, politically.

With the ACA, rather than revolutionizing the system, the federal government chose to make complex additions, subtractions, and other edits to an already complex structure. The system was not gutted or torn down and then rebuilt in a completely rational and solid manner. The ACA reinforces, rather than changes, the fundamental structure of US health insurance, with the nonelderly population being heavily dependent

---

[2] Butler, "Affordable Care Act."

on private health insurance provided by their employer. As a result, the ACA is too complex. There is public confusion about the differences between Medicare, Medicaid, and the ACA; moreover, many Americans do not realize that "Obamacare" is not a synonym for the ACA. Employers, patients, and providers still have to navigate dozens of private and public insurers offering different, ever-changing plans and rules, and obtaining prior approvals for services remains a tedious, time-consuming core feature of health insurance. The Medicaid program and the state insurance exchanges require costly, burdensome means testing.

In the wake of the ACA's adoption, the individual marketplace has not become considerably more competitive. Over time, the ACA's individual market has transformed from an unsubsidized, lightly regulated market to one that contains benefit mandates, pricing restrictions, and high subsidies. It seems that, contrary to what was predicted, competition in the individual market has decreased rather than increased overall. Many current markets are now dominated by a few health care providers, decreasing competition and yielding higher prices, and certain key players in the health care sector (e.g., device makers, drug companies, insurance companies, and specialty physicians) have an exceptionally strong market position.

6.2 Costs for Government, Employers, and Patients under ACA

The ACA has increased the cost of health care and health insurance as the act's Medicaid expansion has proven to be more expensive than projected. Even if all of the cost-saving provisions of the ACA were fully implemented successfully, which they were not, the act was still projected to increase total health spending. The initial ACA portal budget was $93.7 million, but that grew to an ultimate cost of $1.7 billion because of the extensive fixes required.[3] The ACA has reduced the ranks of the uninsured but at a high cost. The percentage of US gross domestic product spent on health care has continued to increase.[4] The bipartisan Congressional Budget Office estimates that, over the next decade, the ACA's expansion and subsidies will cost about $2.5 trillion in total.[5] Also, the US Treasury will lose more than $5.3 trillion given that employer-provided health insurance is tax-free.[6]

The ACA's Medicaid expansion, which is primarily responsible for most of the decline in uninsured Americans, has generated a higher cost than

---

[3] ABC123, "Failed Launch of www.HealthCare.gov."
[4] Madden, "Healthcare Spending Projections." [5] Congressional Budget Office, *Federal Subsidies*.
[6] Congressional Budget Office, *Federal Subsidies*.

anticipated. Unfortunately, the ACA has not fully bent the cost curve down, substantially increased choice, or radically reduced insurance costs. In essence, although there was the best of intentions, the ACA expanded coverage without a corresponding focus on cost containment. The ACA's cost-sharing subsidies, coverage expansion, direct benefits, and premium assistance all worked to raise costs, demand, and utilization for health care in the United States. For example, in the wake of the ACA, emergency room use has remained high.

One beacon of hope is that, while costs continue to rise, they are doing so at a declining rate of growth. Several factors have slowed the rate of health care cost increases, including greater use of electronic medical records, lower health care use during COVID-19, and modulated growth of high-cost medical technologies. The ACA promoted accountable care arrangements where health providers collaborate to manage a patient's health and other cost-saving initiatives. However, the sheer complexity of the US health care system makes it difficult to effectively implement cost-control measures. Yet, universal health care coverage (UHC) in the United States needs to be accompanied by cost containment. If the federal government simply insured everyone under the current system, that would in no way be affordable; the nation would go bankrupt.

For expenditures, there are three faces of evil: **health care abuse**, **health care fraud**, and **health care waste**. There is enrollment fraud related to the ACA, as agents, brokers, lead generators, and enrollees themselves understate income and submit false income verification forms. The administrative costs of private insurance companies include advertising, marketing, sales, providing prior approval, and processing claims. Some recommend that **medical loss ratios** (the proportion of premiums spent on actual care) for payers should be at least 85 percent for group plans and 80 percent for individuals, but this is not easy to enforce. By itself, the ACA has not been able to limit abuse, fraud, and waste; in fact, the ACA has led to growth in improper Medicaid payments to recipients who do not qualify. To address abuse, fraud, and waste, it is important to continue conducting experiments in health care (e.g., accountable care organizations, medical homes, pay-for-performance).

As one of its features, the ACA was going to "bend the cost curve" downward for companies and patients, but health care costs have continued to increase unabated. As shown in Figure 6.1, the average amount spent on premiums by employers and employees has continued to increase.[7]

---

[7] Sarasohn-Kahn, "Health Insurance Premiums."

Employer Premiums and Deductibles Have Risen Much Faster than Wages Since 2010

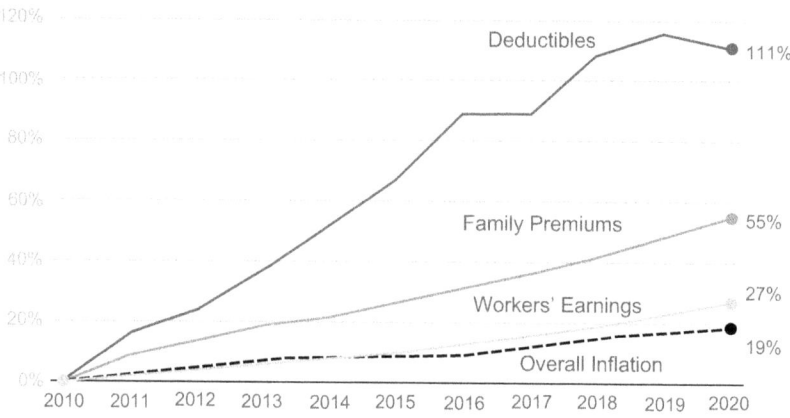

Figure 6.1 Employer premiums, deductibles, and wages since 2010
Source: Kaiser Family Foundation
Note: Average general annual deductibles are for single coverage and are among all covered workers. Workers in plans without a general annual deductible for in-network services are assigned a value of zero.

Premiums for the individual and employer-sponsored markets have increased significantly in many cases. ACA-marketplace enrollees often have to pay high copays, deductibles, and premiums, limiting access to primary care. In some cases, premiums for individual market plans have doubled. Low-income families often choose cheap catastrophic coverage with deductibles so high that use is discouraged. With the ACA in many areas, plan deductibles and premiums soared even as the number of health systems and physicians accepting coverage declined.

One straightforward way to cut costs is to have high-deductible policies that essentially offload costs to sick people. If employers and governments are not required to pay more, then patients either have to pay more or go without certain medical services. Since the ACA's marketplaces came into effect in 2014, several states have taken steps to lower premiums and out-of-pocket costs further for those buying marketplace coverage. Both reinsurance and additional supplemental financial assistance lower the cost to consumers by increasing federal and state health care funding, and by adding covered lives, they improve the risk pool. With reinsurance programs, states (fourteen currently) reimburse insurers for coverage on high-cost marketplace enrollees.[8]

Healthy people are more likely to enroll in insurance if the premiums are more affordable; this improves the risk pool. Yet, as noted earlier, the ratio of healthy/young to sick/old enrollees in the ACA has been lower than expected. One issue is that millions of Americans did have their plans canceled and they lost access to their physicians because their coverage did not meet the ACA rules; this hurt the perception of the ACA brand among the populace.

6.3 Externalities, Incentives, and Outcomes for Patients under ACA

The lack of transparency is one continued issue for the ACA and for the US health care system generally. The pricing for medical care is not transparent to patients or to employers who contract with insurers. As a result, the same procedure, administered in the same geographic area, can vary substantially in price, based on the provider doing the care and the payer covering the cost. In recent years, the federal government has strengthened price transparency rules so that patients and employers can access prices prior to purchasing health care services. These rules empower better individual and organizational consumers of care, and there may be merit to adopting a comprehensive requirement that hospitals and physicians post the prices they charge for basic services (e.g., office visits, elective procedures). Despite the movement to "consumerization" of health care and greater patient centricity, patients rarely have an opportunity to negotiate the price of health care services. Even the employer has limited negotiating leeway, so more companies should consider negotiating directly with providers. Instead, the primary negotiation on price occurs between the provider and the payer; yet, ironically, neither of these two major entities has a consistently strong incentive to control prices.

Adverse selection occurs because the policyholder almost always has better information than insurers regarding their risk levels. As a result, those with a higher degree of risk are likely to find health insurance more attractive, and those with lower risk are likely to find it less attractive. A negative cycle can be created where more and more healthy, low-risk people migrate out of the pool and are replaced by sicker, high-risk people. This undermines desirable risk spreading. Many ACA-exchange plans are Medicaid-based plans offering narrow networks of hospitals and physicians

---

[8] Kaiser Family Foundation, "State Innovation Waivers."

but with lower premiums. Those who are healthy prefer these plans because they are more concerned with having lower premiums than they are with having broader provider networks. Those who are sick prefer a broader choice of providers and more coverage (e.g., for specialty drugs).

Moral hazard refers to the tendency of any insured party to exercise less care or incur more costs when another party (i.e., the insurer) will cover most or even all of those costs. With moral hazard, because insurance coverage lowers the marginal cost of care to the individual, it tends to result in increased health care utilization. The holding of health insurance may even induce some individuals to exert less effort in maintaining their health because health insurance covers some of the financial costs caused by unhealthy behaviors (e.g., poor diet, not exercising, smoking). The ACA also holds the potential to disincentivize workers by discouraging them from taking and continuing full-time jobs because the subsidies for health-exchange plans decrease as household income increases. Expanding the number of insured people tends to make emergency room visits rise, rather than fall, because the newly insured people are less concerned about the cost. Both adverse selection and moral hazard work to increase costs.

Despite its higher cost to the health care system, the ACA has not increased life expectancy. In the pre-adoption decade, life expectancy in the United States increased about 1.5 years per decade, but that positive trend line has ended and even reversed itself. Surprisingly, life expectancy in the United States has been declining in recent years,[9] as captured by Figure 6.2.

Thus, Americans are now dying younger than they were a decade ago, which is contrary to our default expectation of the life expectancy growing monotonically. Within the last decade, life expectancy fell for three consecutive years for the first time in nearly 100 years. The opioid epidemic has likely had a significant effect on the growth of life expectancy, especially when fentanyl flooded US markets in 2015 and beyond, and this crisis was surely not created by the ACA. Other social determinants of health, like housing insecurity, tend to make it harder to be healthy, so the challenge is much bigger than the ACA.

Whenever health care is "free" at the point of service (e.g., as in Canada), demand for that care tends to be quite high. If UHC were ultimately fully successful, the demand for medical care could exceed the supply of care, resulting in increased wait times for appointments, elective surgeries, or other elements. The reason for generally longer wait times in government-run

---

[9] Berg, "Falling U.S. Life Expectancy."

6.3 Externalities, Incentives, and ACA Outcomes

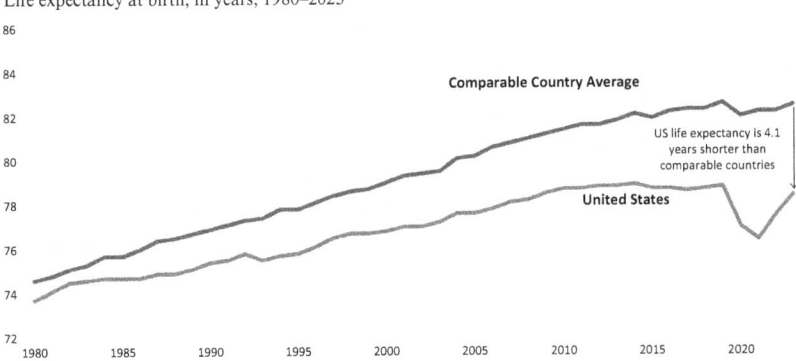

Figure 6.2 Life expectancy
Source: Kaiser Family Foundation analysis of CDC, OECD, Australian Bureau of Statistics, German Federal Statistical Office, Japanese Ministry of Health, Labour, and Welfare, Statistics Canada, and UK Office for National Statistics data.
Notes: Comparable countries include Australia, Austria, Belgium, Canada, France, Germany, Japan, the Netherlands, Sweden, Switzerland, and the UK. The 2023 UK life expectancy data is only for England and Wales. See the "Methods" section of "How does U.S. life expectancy compare to other countries?"

health care systems rests on the basic laws of supply and demand. Amtrak, the US Postal Service, and the VA Health System are vivid examples that show how government-run entities can struggle. Yet, in the United States, underuse is a considerably more common and serious issue than overuse, even with those who are insured. For example, only a small percentage of insured Americans who experience serious symptoms (e.g., chest pains, shortness of breath) see a physician. Even for issues as serious as blocked arteries, gallbladder impairment, unexplained bleeding, and unexplained loss of consciousness, many Americans decline to see a health care professional.

Underuse probably cannot be eliminated or even reduced without spending significantly more money. It can be difficult to reduce overuse by some covered lives while not further suppressing underuse by others. While better population health is definitely good (e.g., if the populace is healthier, labor force participation rates can increase), ironically, longer lifespans could serve to increase health care costs, so one key is to have people live longer lives that are also relatively healthy. Thus, the ACA encounters a buzz saw of complicated issues (e.g., how to increase use by some while decreasing use by others, how to grow coverage while satisfying demand).

6.4 Across the Pond: Externalities and Incentives for Providers and Payers

With decidedly mixed success, the ACA aimed to address a range of externalities and misaligned incentives held by providers and payers; it also created new problems. All things being equal, the private sector is generally more motivated by incentives enabling them to be more profitable. In theory, we want to encourage key health care entities to generate as much value (i.e., ratio of benefits to costs) as possible. Pay for performance offers one prominent pathway that the ACA emphasized. Providers will need to continue taking on more risk for both cost and quality as the pressure grows for value-based care models, including fee-for-value, global capitation, and shared risk. The most common financial incentive is pay for performance. The US system remains primarily a fee-for-service model, which creates a well-documented incentive to do more treatment and do it at higher prices. Pay for performance can sometimes encourage health care providers to shift resources to patients whose care is measured and away from patients whose care is not (e.g., "teaching to the test"). Pay for performance is also challenged by the fact that the ultimate success of treatment is dependent on a variety of factors.

Unfortunately, providers still have some perverse incentives. For example, US health care providers run considerably more diagnostic tests than their counterparts in similar Western countries. With defensive medicine, the physician and health care team are influenced by the potential for a malpractice lawsuit in making decisions about care, diagnosis, and treatment. Practicing defensive medicine can drive up health care costs. This is another case of misaligned incentives. For physicians, who have relatively little incentive to reduce cost and a relatively high incentive to avoid civil litigation, which could be costly in terms of finances and reputation, it is rational to order more rather than fewer tests. Also, some hospitals try to avoid admitting patients who might trigger a readmission penalty and thereby hurt their performance rating.

One counterintuitive example is in the area of prevention, which is generally lauded as positive in health care. Preventive services are typically administered to millions of patients, which costs a significant amount of money, but often prevents disease in only a relatively small subset. Although some preventive services (e.g., mammograms) do save money, many do not.[10] As with all medical care, preventive services are not 100 percent accurate (e.g., false negatives or false positives in cancer

---

[10] Cohen, Neumann, and Weinstein, "Preventive Care."

detection) or 100 percent effective (e.g., flu shots typically work in only about 50 percent of recipients). Frequently, preventive services can cost more to supply than the money they save, raising net costs overall. Preventive care often costs more than it saves because physicians may need to treat many minor conditions in order to prevent one serious health episode. Similarly, several disease management programs do not save money, and because of that, they may actually raise total costs.[11] The goal of disease-management efforts is to stop chronic diseases (e.g., diabetes) from worsening, but many of these ailments are stubbornly resistant to treatment.

Some health insurers may try to frame their plans and prices to attract the healthy and avoid the sick. "Utilization review" involves someone at an insurance company reviewing and then approving/denying a physician's request for some treatment option. As part of what is submitted for review, "upcoding" occurs when Medicare Advantage insurers tell the **Centers for Medicare & Medicaid Services** that their enrollees are sicker than they really are in order to secure higher reimbursement. This upcoding behavior is pursued more aggressively than when physicians treat patients within the traditional Medicare program. Approximately 30 percent of all Medicare beneficiaries are insured via the Medicare Advantage program, which is the privatized branch of Medicare.

6.5 Artificial Intelligence as a Tool for Shaping Health Care Policy

Advances in AI are reshaping health care delivery, but, unfortunately, the ACA was developed just before the proliferation of practical application of AI techniques and tools. With regard to health care, AI holds the potential to help improve quality and lower costs.[12] Due to its combination of massive size and sheer complexity, the US health care system, which totals over $4 trillion, is the one sector that stands to potentially benefit the most from AI. As such, AI presents the rare opportunity to simultaneously expand access to health care services while reducing the burden and costs on the traditional health care system.[13] The utilization of AI is likely to be even more impactful than the average technological "shock" and is already positively impacting the sectors of health care, life sciences, and medicine. Any major future health care legislation needs to put AI at the forefront.

---

[11] Mattke, Seid, and Ma, "Effect of Disease Management."
[12] Harris, Mehrotra, and So, "The Fiscal Frontier."
[13] Harris, Mehrotra, and So, "The Fiscal Frontier."

Along with data and technology, AI represents the most promising pathway to radically improve health care access, affordability, and quality, potentially doing so in a relatively partisan-free manner.

More specifically, AI has the ability to improve diagnostic accuracy and improve patient outcomes while reducing wasteful spending on inappropriate treatments. AI is already beginning to have a positive impact on the major steps of diagnostic care, including receiving input data, medical imagery (e.g., X-rays and MRIs), and physician notes. In terms of diagnosis, AI demonstrates "superhuman performance," usually far exceeding physicians on quality and quantity of analyses. Providers are using AI to attain more accurate diagnoses, personalize treatments, streamline operations, and improve processes in dozens of other key areas. AI is having a positive impact on drug discovery, operational efficiency, and predictive analytics, and it can be used for personalized care plans and patient outreach.

Advances in AI have made cardiac CT less difficult to use, and embedding AI in ultrasound systems allows for better detection, diagnosis, and monitoring of cardiac conditions. By automating and accelerating echocardiographic measurements, AI technologies can rapidly and accurately detect signs of cardiotoxicity much earlier in the treatment process. Using AI in the prevention arena leads to clear cost savings, and its utilization aligns with the incentives of providers and private insurers. Machine learning (ML) is a subset of AI; it leverages vast amounts of data to "learn" and continuously improve its predictive accuracy. It can help analyze and identify patterns in large, complex datasets. For example, by analyzing complex medical imaging data considerably more accurately and quickly than humans can, ML algorithms enable early detection of cancer.

While it is unclear whether the ACA increased, decreased, or had no effect on the number of physicians and other health care professionals,[14] there is an estimated shortage of 200,000–450,000 nurses in the United States[15] and there is predicted to be a continuing shortage of primary-care physicians and medical specialties in future years.[16] With clinical staff stretched thin, health care leaders are utilizing automation to reduce the burden, particularly in terms of relief from repetitive processes and tasks. Appointment scheduling, patient flow management, and preliminary data analysis can all be done by AI programs. Generative, interpretive, and predictive AI can be used to combat clinician burnout, confirm diagnoses,

---

[14] Guth, Garfield, and Rudowitz, "Effects of Medicaid Expansion."
[15] Berlin et al., "Impact of COVID-19."
[16] Association of American Medical Colleges, "Mounting Physician Shortage."

keep patients informed, streamline routine administrative tasks, and transcribe speech/notes. Voice-powered services are becoming increasingly facile at clinical documentation.

Labor-saving AI tools can be leveraged to free up physician time for patient care and other urgent needs. Generative AI can be used to boost clinician productivity via tools such as virtual assistants. Large language models can organize clinical notes and streamline how patient information is communicated across health care teams, and generative AI can translate complex medical information into common terms for patients, allowing for increased engagement. AI can substantially simplify complex diagnoses, allowing less experienced professionals to provide high-quality care with confidence and skill. It is important to note that AI and ML offer the potential to support rather than replace health care professionals.

AI will continue to be a revolutionary, transformative force in health care. By creating more robust pathways for self-management, AI could "democratize" access to the health care system much as the way the internet brought changes to the media sector, making it considerably more grassroots. AI-driven, precision-targeted drug discovery, diagnosis, and treatment require skilled, talented human capital for its development and implementation. There are financial-capital and human-capital needs attendant to AI proliferation. Investment in health care AI is expected to grow significantly over the next few years.[17] Much of this financial fuel will be provided by angel investors, family offices, investment banking, private equity, and venture capital. It is hard to pick out which companies and technologies will prove to be "winners" and which ones will ultimately fail to gain traction, but we are on the cusp of a technological revolution. Significant training, reskilling, and partnering will be needed to address the current shortage of AI expertise in health care. Now and for the foreseeable future, AI will require humans.

Blockchain technology serves as a highly complementary companion to AI. Companies can use these technologies to improve inventory management, including minimizing demand fluctuations, disruptions, and fraud. AI, ML, and blockchain technology are helping to overhaul the drug and medical supply chains, substantially improving transparency and traceability. As data breaches and other hacks continue to increase in frequency and severity, AI will play a crucial role in cybersecurity as it can help prevent, detect, and mitigate attacks in real time.

AI in health care is viewed with enthusiasm/optimism by some and despair/fear by others. As with much of health care, there are some barriers regarding

---

[17] Medical Group Management Association, "Ambient Technology's Role."

bureaucracy, incentive misalignment, and regulations. For example, in terms of incentives, AI could serve to diagnose more items needing treatment, which would ironically increase costs in that regard. That dulls the incentives of some insurers to encourage AI adoption for diagnosis. Some are concerned that AI is an immature technology that could do harm to patients. Despite these misgivings, we should also be mindful of the harm we could cause by delaying implementation. Public–private partnerships will be essential to driving a successful rollout of AI across health care.

Chapter Summary

The ACA represents a complex and significant shift in the landscape of American health care. While it has successfully reduced the number of uninsured individuals through its provisions, such as community ratings and guaranteed issue, the overall effectiveness is questionable in some areas, especially regarding cost containment. The initial rollout was marred by technical failures and a slow adoption rate, leading enrollment figures to fall short of projections, with the biggest gaps being among the young and healthy. Furthermore, the ACA's reliance on Medicaid expansion raises concerns about the sustainability of services for other vulnerable populations, revealing the intricate trade-offs that accompany nationwide health care reform. Despite the ACA's good intentions to control costs, overall health care spending has continued to rise, and the anticipated competition in the individual insurance market failed to materialize the robust level of savings that was anticipated.

The complexities of the ACA, coupled with public confusion regarding different insurance programs, have created barriers for consumers seeking affordable care. Additionally, issues such as adverse selection and moral hazard have further complicated effectiveness. Looking forward, AI and blockchain technology represent opportunities to address some of these systemic challenges. By enhancing diagnostic accuracy, improving transparency, and streamlining operations, these technologies offer robust potential to foster a more effective, efficient, and equitable health care system. However, successful integration must involve ongoing collaboration between public and private sectors, including patients, providers, payers, and policy makers. Ultimately, the ACA laid a foundation for future reforms, but it also highlights the need for continued innovation and smart policymaking in the pursuit of a health care system that is accessible, affordable, and sustainable for all Americans.

CHAPTER 7

The Health Care Debate: Is It Too Focused on Insurance?

Insights

- Addressing health care costs is necessary but insufficient; policy must also tackle social determinants to close health disparities.
- Factors like housing, education, and food access impact health equity more than solely obtaining access to medical services.
- Treating food, housing, and education as integral to health policy can significantly improve outcomes and reduce disparities.
- Effective health care reform requires addressing systemic barriers like income inequality and geographic disparities in resource distribution.
- Integrating health policy across sectors like housing and education is essential for comprehensive health equity solutions.

The payers are often at the center of the health care debate. This is captured in debates on health care worldwide with "insurance for all" being a common and regularly contentious theme in dialogue. The focus on payers largely comes down to the imminent need to cover costs. How can one access a health care system they can't afford? "Follow the money" is a common phrase that applies to this situation. After all, the path to affordable care more often than not runs through the insurers or payers of that care.

In his timeless book *How to Win Friends and Influence People*, Dale Carnegie recalls a story highlighting the cleverness of Andrew Carnegie, who, while born into poverty, rose to be among the richest Americans in history. In the story, he recalls Andrew's sister-in-law worried about her boys who were attending college. She sent them many letters, but they never replied. Perplexed, Andrew bet her $100 that he could get her boys to reply to him. After someone took his bet, he went ahead and wrote them a letter. As described by Dale Carnegie: "[Andrew Carnegie] wrote his nephews a chatty letter, mentioning casually in a post-script that he was sending each one a five-dollar bill. He neglected, however, to enclose the money. Back came replies by return mail thanking 'Dear Uncle Andrew' for his kind note and ... you can finish the sentence yourself."[1]

Of course, as you can imagine, his nephews reminded him that he "forgot" to include the money. Andrew Carnegie astutely knew to appeal to the interests of his nephews. Similarly, at the forefront of the interests of patients is money (i.e., their ability to pay for their care). Especially in the United States, the costs of health care can be expensive, and if left to citizens to cover those costs without insurance, it can be a significant barrier for tens of millions of people. Addressing costs, then, is naturally a primary concern.

In this chapter, though, we pivot toward a broader conversation on equity. In Chapter 1, we opened with a discussion on health equity using an example to illustrate that getting someone to a doctor is *necessary, but not sufficient* to achieving health equity. Even if we address costs to ensure that all people can afford their care, access to a health care system alone does not necessarily translate into health equity within that system. Expanding the health care debate to be inclusive of the social determinants of health (SDOH) is therefore a necessary next step. Closing health disparities means *meeting people where they are* – which is where about 80 percent of factors that predict their quality of life and length of life interact.[2] Addressing social determinants in health care policy can move the United States toward policy that is both *necessary and sufficient* to meaningfully and comprehensively close health disparity gaps.

7.1 Health Equity and the Social Determinants of Health

Equity may be among the greatest challenges facing health care policy reform in that addressing it requires policies that *meet people where they are*. To explain, consider that the front lines of receiving care typically occur in physician or medical settings (e.g., seeing a doctor for routine care, or visiting an urgent care facility for an immediate medical need). Here, patients can be seen, diagnosed, and cared for. Having access to care, then, allows us to *be healthy*. However, care often extends into the home, where disparities in health equity are the greatest. The front lines of health

---

[1] Carnegie, *How to Win Friends*, 25.
[2] U.S. Department of Health and Human Services, *Healthy People 2030*.

equity occur in the very places where people live, work, and age. Here, factors such as the walkability and safety of our neighborhoods, the viability of transportation, the quality of schools, and access to healthy foods affect our ability to live a healthy lifestyle. Closing disparities in health equity, then, allows us to *live healthy*.

Health equity is the custom distribution of resources to uniquely address inequality in a health care system for each individual. Demographic factors, such as socioeconomic status, race, ethnicity, or geographic location, should not determine health outcomes. Health equity signifies that health is a fundamental human right whereby addressing it can not only improve individual well-being but also enhance collective public health outcomes, leading to a healthier population overall. It inherently recognizes that inequitable distribution of resources can adversely affect health, and by extension, perpetuate disadvantages, particularly in underserved and marginalized communities.

Health equity is strongly linked to **SDOH**, which are the lived environments where people are born, live, learn, work, play, worship, and age that can affect the health of an individual or population.[3] The Commission on Social Determinants of Health (CSDH) at the World Health Organization (WHO) developed a conceptual framework for understanding the impact of SDOH on health equity and well-being. This framework, in Figure 7.1, is particularly useful for considering the potential role of policy to address SDOH. It illustrates how social, economic, and political systems create socioeconomic levels from which populations are stratified by psychosocial and demographic factors. This stratification, in turn, influences specific determinants of health that are indicative of an individual's position or status within social structures.

The conceptual framework for the SDOH developed by the CSDH is a structured approach, aimed at addressing health inequities through a better understanding of the underlying social, economic, and political factors that influence health outcomes. It serves as a guide for policy makers to identify effective interventions to combat health disparities. It further recognizes that the relationship between SDOH and one's health is reciprocal. For example, people can face differing levels of exposure to and risk of health-related issues, which can, in turn, impact their social status, such as their job opportunities or income. Likewise, on a larger scale, widespread diseases, such as COVID-19, can disrupt the functioning of social, economic, and political institutions.

---

[3] U.S. Department of Health and Human Services, *Social Determinants of Health*.

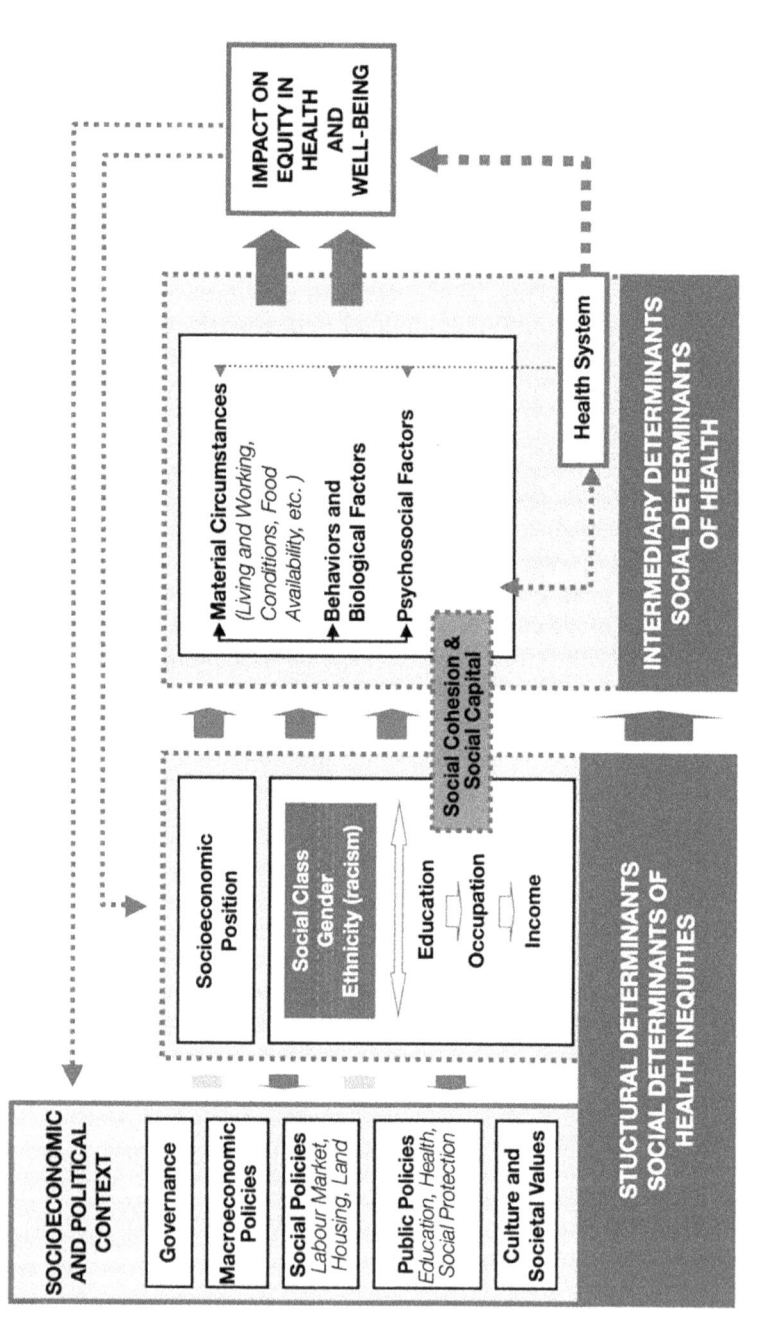

Figure 7.1 The CSDH conceptual framework for the social determinants of health

Source: Solar O, Irwin A. A conceptual framework for action on the social determinants of health. 2010. Social Determinants of Health Discussion Paper 2 (Policy and Practice), p. 6. Geneva, Switzerland: World Health Organization. License: CC BY-NC-SA 3.0 IGO.

The framework consists of three core components: socioeconomic and political context, structural determinants of health inequities, and intermediary determinants of health. The *socioeconomic and political context* includes the overarching societal structures that create stratification and influence individuals' socioeconomic positions. Factors such as education, income, and social class play critical roles in shaping health outcomes. The *structural determinants* are the social and political mechanisms that generate inequalities, while the *intermediary determinants* are the direct factors impacting health, such as housing and access to health care services. Understanding the disconnect between these two types of determinants is crucial for effective interventions.

A critical aspect of the CSDH framework is the differentiation between structural and intermediary determinants of health. Structural determinants encompass broad societal mechanisms that produce social hierarchies, such as income distribution and educational opportunities. In contrast, intermediary determinants are more immediate factors that directly affect health, including living conditions, behavioral patterns, and the quality of health care services.

7.2 The Social Determinants and Health Policy

The conceptual framework developed by the CSDH reveals that the SDOH have inherent political implications, resulting in a proposed framework for leveraging policy to address health inequities driven by the SDOH, as summarized in Figure 7.2. Effective actions consequently require a commitment from policy makers to address the structural and social issues that can perpetuate inequity. Let's consider seven implications of this framework to reveal the dynamic relationship between politics, power dynamics, and health outcomes:

1. *Inherently political nature of health interventions.* Health interventions targeting social determinants are not merely technical or medical solutions, but, rather, they involve complex societal changes. These interventions often confront the existing power structures and resource distributions, making them inherently political.
2. *Power relations and health equity.* The framework recognizes that health inequities are often a result of unequal power distribution in society. Addressing these inequities can require, to some extent, a redistribution of power, resources, and opportunities, which is fundamentally a political process.

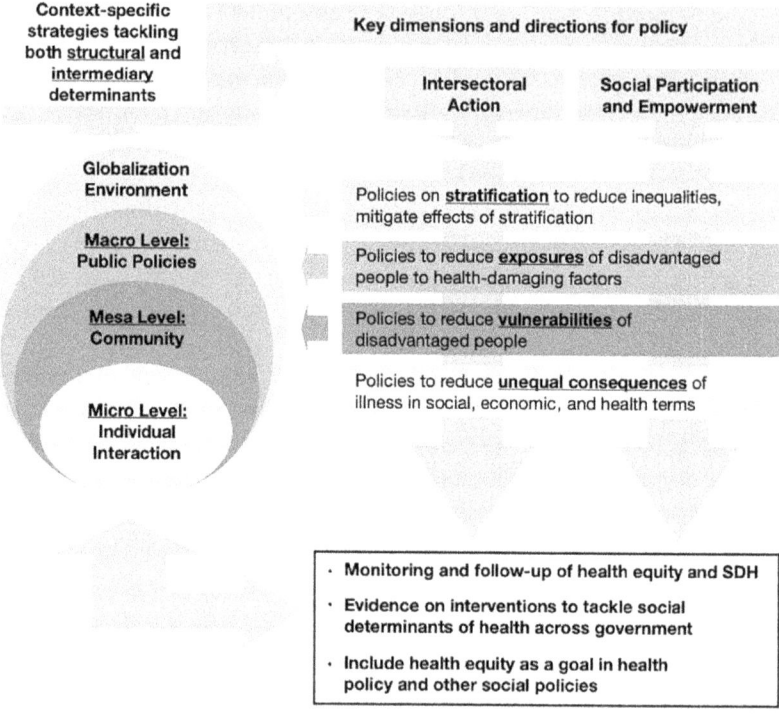

Figure 7.2 The CSDH conceptual framework for addressing health inequities
Source: Solar O, Irwin A. A conceptual framework for action on the social determinants of health. 2010. Social Determinants of Health Discussion Paper 2 (Policy and Practice), p. 8. Geneva, Switzerland: World Health Organization. License: CC BY-NC-SA 3.0 IGO.

3. *Role of policy makers.* Policy makers play a crucial role in addressing structural issues that perpetuate health inequities. This involves:
   - recognizing the political nature of health interventions,
   - committing to potentially unpopular or challenging policy changes, and
   - addressing root causes rather than just symptoms of health inequities.
4. *Structural issues and health.* Structural issues refer to systemic factors like economic policies, education systems, and social norms that shape health outcomes. These issues are deeply embedded in societal structures and require long-term, sustained efforts to change.

5. *Systematic advocacy.* The framework emphasizes the need for organized, persistent advocacy efforts. This involves:
   - building coalitions among diverse stakeholders,
   - educating the public and decision-makers about SDOH, and
   - pushing for evidence-based policies that address root causes of health inequities.
6. *Policy changes for equitable health outcomes.* The ultimate goal is to implement policies that promote health equity across all population groups. This may include:
   - universal health care access,
   - addressing income inequality,
   - improving education and employment opportunities, and
   - enhancing social protection measures.
7. *Challenges and resistance.* Efforts to shift power relations and implement structural changes often face resistance from those benefiting from the status quo. Overcoming this resistance requires sustained political will and public support.

The CSDH framework underscores the idea that improving population health is not just a matter of medical interventions. It is a complex, multifaceted effort involving social, economic, and political transformations that requires a holistic approach to address health inequities through political action and policy reform. Policy makers must recognize that access to point of care ("insurance for all") is a first step, and not *the* step to close health equity gaps. Achieving health equity requires considerate policy that extends beyond the point of care.

7.3 Thinking beyond the Point of Care

While access to health care is undeniably important, it is not sufficient on its own to ensure optimal health. The SDOH encompass a wide range of factors that can influence health outcomes, including socioeconomic status, education, and the environment.[4] These determinants contribute to health inequities such that merely having access to health care does not necessarily equate to positive health outcomes.

---

[4] U.S. Centers for Disease Control and Prevention, *Social Determinants of Health*.

Environmental conditions, for example, have a significant impact on health. Poor air quality is linked to respiratory diseases, cardiovascular problems, and higher rates of mortality.[5] Water quality significantly affects health outcomes, with contaminated drinking water leading to waterborne diseases like cholera, diarrhea, and typhoid.[6] Living conditions significantly impact health, with individuals in low-income neighborhoods having poorer health outcomes, including cardiovascular disease and respiratory issues, in part, due to limited access to exercise, healthy food options, transportation, and safety.[7] Likewise, the choices we make, such as our diet and physical activity, significantly contribute to our length of life and quality of life. Still more factors, such as workplace stress (e.g., hours worked per week, demands in the workplace) and family dynamics (e.g., acceptance and support from family members), can impact our health. Therefore, access to a physician or to medical services is necessary, but it is not sufficient to ensure optimal health outcomes. Even those with health care access may experience adverse health outcomes due to a variety of factors *outside* the health care system itself, which, at a policy level, means we need to think beyond "insurance for all" to meet people where they are, literally.

A point of evidence that underpins the need for health policy that extends beyond the point of care or "insurance for all" is **medication adherence**, which is the extent to which a person's actions correspond with or follow the agreed-upon recommendations from a health care provider.[8] Certainly, factors within the health care system that can improve medication adherence include simplifying the complexity of medication schedules, especially those for multiple chronic conditions, reducing the cost of therapies and medications, and improving patient education at the point of service. However, many more factors beyond the health care system also impact medication adherence. Economic affluence and stability, for example, with those from more affluent and stable regions (e.g., those earning greater income, those from households with two parents, and those with greater housing stability) showing increased rates of medication adherence.[9] Other examples include education and health literacy, access to health care services (including costs, transportation, and availability of providers), social support (from family, friends, and community members to help manage patient health), and food and housing insecurity.

---

[5] U.S. Environmental Protection Agency, *Particle Pollution*.
[6] U.S. Centers for Disease Control and Prevention, *Global Water*.
[7] U.S. Centers for Disease Control and Prevention, *Socioeconomic Factors*.
[8] Dobbels et al., "Growing Pains."   [9] Truveta Research, "SDOH Factors."

A broader concern is the structure of health care in the United States, which is largely designed under the assumption that patients lead middle-class lives. In his TEDMED talk, Dr. Mitchell Katz critiques the US health care system's built-in assumptions, which often do not align with the realities of low-income patients' lives.[10] He argues from firsthand experience that the system operates with a "middle-class model" that inadvertently excludes or complicates access for the most vulnerable populations. Key assumptions highlighted in his talk include the belief that patients have:

- A stable home environment, including access to a refrigerator (essential for medications like insulin), a bathroom, and a secure place to rest.
- The ability to speak and understand English, which affects comprehension of medical instructions and engagement with health care providers.
- Flexible work schedules, allowing them to attend appointments or receive care during traditional business hours.
- Access to a working telephone, which health care providers rely on for contact and follow-up care.
- Sufficient and steady food supplies to support medication regimens and recovery.

A key takeaway that has implications for effectively implementing universal health care[11] is that many assumptions made in the US health care system are factors that occur outside the system itself. In other words, at a provider level, US health care can often be designed in ways that contribute to disparities by not being adaptive to the SDOH that impact not only the ability for people to *be* healthy but also their ability to *live* a healthy lifestyle. These assumptions exacerbate health care disparities, as they can prevent low-income individuals from effectively accessing and adhering to health care recommendations, which highlights the need for health care policies that adapt to varied social and economic realities to improve inclusivity and equity in patient care.

7.4 Examples of Policy in the United States and Abroad

The focus on SDOH reflects a need to consider more than the point of care where patients receive services. With nearly 80 percent of length-of-life and quality-of-life measures predicted by factors outside the health care system, it is critical to be considerate of *where* people live and *how* they live their

---

[10] Katz, "US Healthcare System."   [11] Das et al., "Rethinking Assumptions."

lives. In the United States, the Affordable Care Act (ACA) was a positive step toward addressing SDOH. Examples of how the ACA addresses SDOH include:

- National Prevention Council and Strategy: The ACA established the National Prevention Council, which is composed of leaders from twenty federal departments and agencies who collectively develop a National Prevention Strategy. This strategy aims to enhance the health of Americans by addressing key social and environmental factors that influence health outcomes.
- Expansion of Medicaid: The ACA expanded Medicaid eligibility to include individuals and families with incomes up to 138 percent of the federal poverty level. This expansion increases access to health care services for low-income individuals, mitigating the impact of socioeconomic factors associated with health disparities.
- Community Health Centers Funding: The ACA increased funding for community health centers, which are vital for providing care to underserved populations. These centers serve as crucial access points for primary care, helping to address barriers related to access to transportation and health services.
- Accountable Health Communities Model: Under the ACA, the Center for Medicare and Medicaid Innovation introduced the Accountable Health Communities model, which connects Medicare and Medicaid beneficiaries with community services to address health-related social needs. This initiative aims to improve health outcomes by recognizing the influence of social factors such as food insecurity, housing, and transportation.

Internationally, various countries have implemented public health policies that target SDOH to improve health equity. Some examples from the international public health policies include:

- Universal Health Coverage in South Africa: In South Africa, the government implemented a policy that offers free retroviral therapy to all HIV-positive patients, regardless of their income or health status. This policy aims to improve health equity, especially for Black populations disproportionately affected by HIV, significantly reducing annual mortality rates among these individuals.
- Early Childhood Development Policies in the WHO European Region: The WHO promotes policies focused on early childhood development, such as providing early childhood education. This

initiative is designed to reduce achievement gaps, improve health outcomes, and support health equity among children from low-income families.
- Free Health Services in Thailand: Thailand's Universal Coverage Scheme provides free health services to all citizens, specifically targeting lower-income populations. The program aims to alleviate the financial burden of health care and promote equal access to necessary health services, thereby addressing economic and social barriers to health care.
- Health Promotion Campaigns in Australia: Australia implements wide-ranging health promotion campaigns aimed at reducing smoking rates and encouraging healthy eating among disadvantaged communities. These campaigns are designed to address specific lifestyle factors that contribute to health disparities among lower socioeconomic groups, promoting healthier behaviors and environments.

These examples illustrate comprehensive efforts made in the United States and internationally, through policy, to address various dimensions of SDOH with the aim to improve overall health equity and outcomes. Efforts to close healthy equity gaps must go beyond the point of care to address the SDOH that account for about 80 percent of length of life and quality of life.[12] The idea that insurance for all solves the health care crisis in the United States is simply misguided. Insurance for all is necessary, but not sufficient to optimize a health care system that is accessible to all in a way that is equitable for all.

In November 2023, the White House released the fifty-three-page *U.S. Playbook to Address Social Determinants of Health*, stating that "Improving health and well-being across America requires addressing the social circumstances and related environmental hazards and exposures that improve health outcomes."[13] For a long time, many in academia have argued that boosting public investment in social services might lower and prevent health care expenses. Notably, while the United States spends more on health care than other industrialized nations, it spends substantively less on social services (about 16 percent vs. 20 percent of GDP, respectively).

One challenge for balancing reimbursement across health care and social services is the structure for funding US health care. In the *Playbook*, it identifies that "funds associated with 'health' are too often walled off from investments in improving SDOH." In other words, too often, those

---

[12] National Committee for Quality Assurance (NCQA), "Health Equity."
[13] Domestic Policy Council, *Social Determinants of Health*.

investing in SDOH do not have access to reimbursement or funding dedicated to "health care" services. Other SDOH advocates cite a **wrong pockets problem**, in which one entity makes investments to improve a social condition while another entity accrues the benefits. To address this, it is critical to be considerate of how returns on investment are split between public and private sectors, or between public agencies.[14,15] For example, the federal government could see savings in reduced Medicare costs through infrastructure spending by states.

The following are a few practical ways the United States can strengthen health care policy by focusing more on the SDOH:

- Broadening care to include nonmedical factors. Health Care policies typically focus on clinical care (at the point of care) rather than addressing also the broader social, economic, and environmental factors influencing health outcomes. Broadening the focus in policy to be inclusive of nonmedical factors means that vital drivers of health, such as education, income, housing conditions, and transportation, are part of a coordinated, equitable solution for health.
- Integrating the SDOH in health care delivery. Many health care systems lack the infrastructure (e.g., data systems, workflows, and provider trainings) to incorporate SDOH into patient care effectively.[16] Despite evidence that addressing social needs can lead to better health outcomes, policies frequently do not mandate the assessment of social determinants in clinical settings, thereby missing opportunities to connect patients with necessary resources.
- Aligning equity with access to care. Access to quality health care is often influenced by socioeconomic status, yet policies often fail to address barriers faced by underserved populations. For example, low-income individuals and those from rural settings tend to have less access to health care services, leading to greater health disparities. This inequity is compounded by insufficient funding for community health workers who could bridge gaps in care.
- Increasing investment in social services. The United States spends significantly more on medical services compared to social services. The **Organisation for Economic Co-operation and Development (OECD)** countries spend about $1.70 on social services for each $1 on health services, on average, whereas the United States spends only

---

[14] Butler, "'Wrong Pockets' Hurt Health."   [15] Butler, "Optimizing Investment in Housing."
[16] Kreuter et al., "Addressing Social Needs."

$0.56 per health dollar, on average.[17] This relative underinvestment in social services makes it difficult to improve health indicators, as effective interventions to promote health equity often lie in enhancing social conditions, such as housing stability and food security.
- Coordinating policy efforts across sectors. Health Care policies do not typically incorporate frameworks that address SDOH across different government sectors like education, housing, and criminal justice. The siloed nature of policymaking makes it difficult to coordinate comprehensive approaches that are capable of meaningfully closing health equity gaps.
- Incorporating behavioral health in health care policy. Many policies neglect the importance of mental health as a critical factor of overall health and largely ignore how socioeconomic factors, like poverty and food insecurity, can influence mental health. This oversight in policy can hinder the effectiveness of health care interventions aimed at improving health outcomes.
- Improving support for prevention programs. Preventive health programs that could mitigate the adverse effects of SDOH are often underfunded. Policies prioritizing treatment over prevention fail to acknowledge the importance of addressing the root causes of health issues, such as poor nutrition and lack of physical activity linked to environmental factors. Preventative care can also be cost-saving to patients and providers, although this can depend on the type of preventative care provided.[18]
- Enhancing responsiveness to racial and ethnic disparities. Policies often fail to specifically target the unique SDOH challenges faced by racial and ethnic minorities, such as historical and systemic racism. Without targeted interventions, these groups continue to experience disproportionately poor health outcomes in comparison to their nonminority counterparts.

To strengthen US health care policy and improve health outcomes, a greater focus on SDOH is essential. This involves expanding health care policy to address nonmedical factors like education, housing, and transportation while integrating SDOH into care delivery through better infrastructure, training, and workflows. Equity must be prioritized to improve access for underserved populations and policies need to be

---

[17] Butler, "Social Spending."
[18] Cohen, Neumann, and Weinstein, "Does Preventive Care Save Money?"

coordinated across sectors to address systemic gaps and include behavioral health as a critical component. Additionally, prioritizing prevention programs and targeting racial and ethnic disparities are vital for fostering health equity. By addressing these interconnected factors, US health care policy can progress toward a more equitable and effective system for all.

7.5 Across the Pond: What Is Medicine?

One critical step toward addressing SDOH in health policy is to recognize the social determinants as "medicine" insofar as they alleviate illness and promote health. In the United States, *medicine* primarily refers to drugs defined by the Food and Drug Administration (FDA) under the Federal Food, Drug, and Cosmetic Act. According to this statute, drugs are articles intended for use in the diagnosis, cure, mitigation, treatment, or prevention of disease in humans or animals.[19] This legal framework ensures that substances classified as medicine undergo rigorous testing for safety and efficacy prior to public use.

Several categories of substances are recognized as medicine, including prescription drugs (e.g., medications that require a doctor's prescription), over-the-counter drugs (e.g., medications that can be purchased without a prescription and are widely available in pharmacies and stores), and biologics (e.g., products derived from living organisms, which can include vaccines, blood products, and gene therapies). Categories that fall outside the definition of medicine in the United States include dietary supplements (e.g., vitamins, minerals, herbs, and amino acids), homeopathic products (e.g., those made from highly diluted substances based on the principle of "like cures like"), and herbal remedies (e.g., plant-based products and formulations). The distinction between what is considered medicine and what is not is crucial for regulatory, legal, and ethical reasons. The courts have often been involved in defining and interpreting the scope of medicine in the United States, especially in complex cases like FDA regulation of reproductive health drugs.

Viewing the SDOH as a driver for health equity requires a policy that integrates these factors into the medicine model. As one example, food is increasingly recognized as a form of medicine in both the United States and OECD nations, particularly through initiatives focused on nutrition and chronic disease management. However, the regulatory frameworks and insurance coverage for food as medicine vary widely. In the United

---

[19] U.S. Food and Drug Administration, "Procedures for Drug Applications."

States, food is increasingly seen as an integral part of health care, with growing initiatives to treat food as medicine. This perspective is gaining traction due to the prevalence of diet-related chronic diseases such as obesity, diabetes, and cardiovascular diseases. The "Food is Medicine" initiative, developed by the Department of Health and Human Services, aims to integrate nutrition into health care delivery by advocating for access to healthy foods and diet-related resources as part of standard medical care.[20] Moreover, proposals such as the National Food as Medicine Program Act, introduced in 2024, intend to expand coverage of food and nutrition programs through health care systems, signifying a legislative push to establish food as a formal component of health care.[21] Research further underscores the efficacy of certain food interventions, such as medically tailored meals, in improving health outcomes and reducing health care costs, although integration into the health care system remains inconsistent and challenges persist regarding insurance coverage for these services.[22]

In OECD countries, food is also increasingly viewed as a crucial element of health care. Many countries have implemented national action plans focusing on the promotion of healthier diets and physical activity as part of their public health strategies. The OECD underscores the importance of addressing poor diets and their associated health risks as part of its efforts to mitigate chronic diseases like obesity and diabetes. For instance, many member countries are already implementing food labeling, lifestyle counseling, and policies that encourage access to healthier food options, aligning with the food-as-medicine concept. While the conceptualization of food as medicine is still evolving in both the US and OECD nations, concrete steps are being taken to integrate these ideas into health care practices.

More broadly, the SDOH, as a whole, are increasingly recognized as critical factors influencing health outcomes, and there is a growing discourse around treating them as integral components of health care. National health frameworks, such as Healthy People 2030 in the United States, explicitly prioritize SDOH as a focal point for improving public health and health equity. This initiative sets data-driven objectives aimed at increasing awareness of SDOH and promoting strategies to mitigate their negative impacts on health.[23] This reflects a shift in the health care community toward recognizing that addressing SDOH can significantly enhance health outcomes and promote health equity.

[20] Office of Disease Prevention and Health Promotion, *Food Is Medicine.*
[21] Totz, "Food as Medicine."
[22] Center for Health Law and Policy Innovation, "Food Is Medicine."
[23] U.S. Centers for Disease Control and Prevention, *Social Determinants of Health.*

Despite the growing recognition of SDOH in the context of health care, challenges remain. Many health care professionals express concerns about their capacity to address SDOH effectively, citing a lack of training and resources.[24] There is also an ongoing debate about how to fund and implement SDOH-related interventions within existing health care systems, particularly in terms of insurance coverage and reimbursement for services that address these determinants. Thus, while there is considerable momentum in framing SDOH as components of health and medicine, substantial work remains if we are to fully integrate these concepts into clinical practices and health policies. The recognition of SDOH as medicine reflects a paradigm shift in the health care landscape, emphasizing the need for a holistic approach to health that transcends traditional medical interventions.

Chapter Summary

The health care debate must be broadened, expanding beyond the narrow focus on insurance and access to care, to address the SDOH that significantly shape health outcomes. While ensuring universal insurance is necessary, it is not sufficient to achieve health equity or improve public health on a meaningful scale. True equity requires addressing the social, economic, and environmental factors that account for nearly 80 percent of quality-of-life and life-expectancy measures. Policies must move beyond the clinical point of care to integrate nonmedical factors like housing stability, education, and access to healthy food, ensuring resources reach individuals where they live and work.

Achieving this vision will require sustained commitment from policy makers, health care providers, and communities to embrace a holistic approach that tackles both structural and intermediary determinants of health. Drawing lessons from international models and leveraging frameworks like the WHO's CSDH, the United States must implement coordinated, equity-driven policies that break down silos between health care and social services. By aligning investments in social services with health care outcomes, addressing systemic disparities, and incorporating behavioral and preventive health measures, the health care system can be transformed, promoting equity and well-being for all. This shift is not merely an enhancement of care delivery – it is a fundamental redefinition of health policy to ensure a healthier, more equitable future.

---

[24] Magnan, "Social Determinants of Health."

CHAPTER 8

Health Equity: Is It Even Possible?

Insights

- Policies must go beyond insurance access to address systemic barriers like housing, food security, and education.
- Marginalized groups face structural discrimination in health care, affecting access, quality of care, and health outcomes.
- Tailored, community-based interventions improve access and trust, addressing the diverse needs of underserved populations.
- Countries with universal health care demonstrate improved access, better preventative care, and reduced disparities compared to fragmented US systems.
- Combining health policies with housing and education, as seen in Scandinavia, reduces disparities and promotes equitable outcomes.

To close health disparity gaps, policies must be considerate of the barriers that prevent people not only from *seeing a doctor* (insurance for all) but also from *living healthy lives* (social determinants). Focusing on *health equity* (defined in Chapter 7) in health care policy is critical to ensuring that every individual – from all walks of life – has a fair and just opportunity to attain their highest level of health, which includes access to both the health care system itself, and access to the resources and services that are necessary to promote their well-being, where they live. Achieving health equity, therefore, requires policy efforts to address inequalities that can create barriers to health care, thereby fostering a more equitable distribution of health outcomes across different population segments.[1]

In an effort to improve health equity, the Affordable Care Act (ACA), for example, expanded access to health insurance by creating marketplaces for affordable coverage, providing subsidies based on income, and

[1] Office of Disease Prevention and Health Promotion, *Healthy People 2030*.

expanding Medicaid eligibility in participating states. Although, due to a variety of factors, this policy was never given a chance to fully roll out, its aim was to reduce the uninsured rate, particularly among low-income individuals, racial and ethnic minorities, and people in rural populations, thereby addressing disparities in access to health care. Efforts to address social determinants in policy also exist internationally. As one example, the National Health Service (NHS), which was established in July 1948 in the United Kingdom, provides universal health care and is funded through taxation. It ensures that all residents, regardless of income or social status, have access to necessary medical services without direct out-of-pocket costs. This model significantly reduces health disparities and promotes equitable access to care across socioeconomic groups.

Meeting people where they are is essential to closing health equity gaps, as it acknowledges and addresses the unique barriers individuals face in accessing health care and achieving well-being. As illustrated in Figure 8.1, Healthy People 2030 provides a framework for leveraging data across leading health indicators to generate collaborative, bipartisan efforts to address the social determinants of health (SDOH) and achieve health equity.[2] By tailoring policies and interventions to account for diverse social, economic, and cultural contexts, we can promote health equity by bridging the gaps in access to care and addressing the underlying social determinants that shape health outcomes. In this chapter, we posit that health equity is not only possible, but that the changes needed to get there are very much achievable.

8.1 Barriers to Health Equity

Addressing health equity in the United States requires a comprehensive understanding of multiple barriers that contribute to disparities in health outcomes across diverse populations. Recall from Figure 1.1 in Chapter 1, we opened by acknowledging that factors outside the health care system (i.e., factors beyond the point of care) account for about 80 percent of length-of-life and quality-of-life measures. In other words, inequities with the SDOH can have a substantive impact on health disparities. In this section, we evaluate health disparities through the lens of systemic inequities, access to health care, and the broader social determinants that affect our health.

---

[2] Office of Disease Prevention and Health Promotion, *Healthy People 2030*.

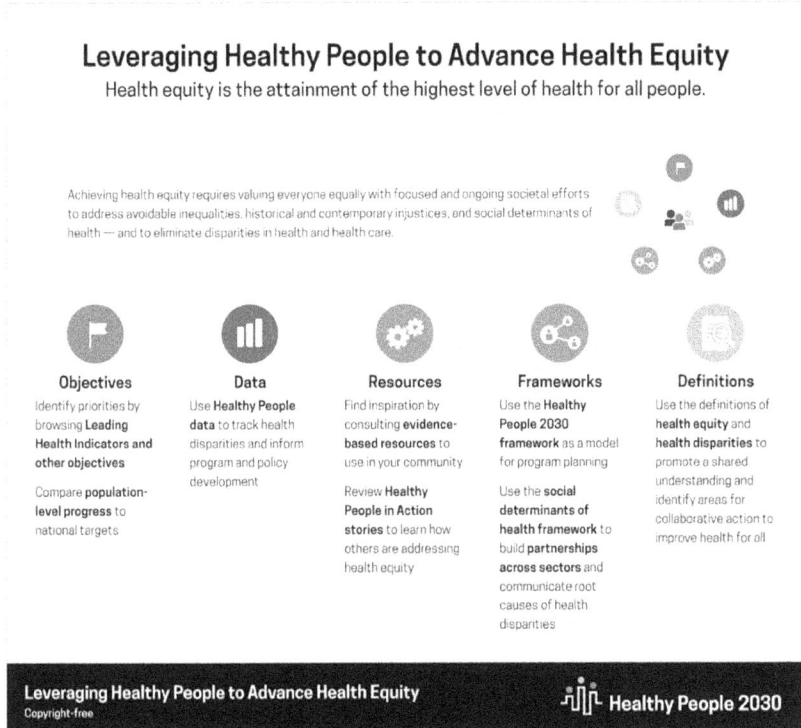

Figure 8.1 Leveraging healthy people to advance health equity
Source: Healthy People 2030

Systemic Inequities

Systemic barriers, often ingrained in organizations, include obstacles, regulations, and structures that deny people or groups access to resources and opportunities that are necessary for their complete engagement in society. These barriers, whether intentional or not, are reflected in policies and practices that have historically marginalized certain groups. These systemic barriers reflect the societal structures that limit access to care for marginalized groups. Policies and practices that have historically marginalized racial and ethnic minorities can contribute to disparities in access to health care, quality of services received, and overall health outcomes.[3] For example, Black and Hispanic populations are less likely to have health insurance and are more likely to endure delays in receiving necessary

---

[3] Radley et al., "Advancing Racial Equity."

medical care due to systemic discrimination. This systemic barrier helps to explain why ending the continuous enrollment for Medicaid and the Children's Health Insurance Program during the pandemic was shown to widen disparities, particularly in marginalized communities like Black and Hispanic populations, who historically have higher uninsured rates.[4]

While we can certainly debate the root causes of such disparities, evidence is clear that patients of color frequently experience interpersonal racism and prejudice in health care settings, and they frequently receive subpar treatment compared to White patients.[5,6,7] The federal Agency for Health Care Research and Quality found that for 52 percent of quality indicators in 2023, Black patients experienced inferior care compared to White patients.[8] Significant differences in both patient safety and quality of care were also discovered in relation to surgery,[9] pain management,[10] maternal health outcomes,[11] and with respect to cancer, stroke, and heart disease.[12]

Disparities in medication prescriptions are well-documented and reflect various systemic issues in health care access and treatment. Black and Hispanic Medicare beneficiaries, for example, use significantly fewer medications than their White counterparts, even when suffering from similar chronic conditions like diabetes and hypertension.[13] In studies focusing on opioid prescriptions, Black and Hispanic patients were less likely than White patients to receive prescriptions of opioid medications for pain management, even for similar levels of pain and with comparable clinical conditions,[14] they were more likely to use the emergency department for pain treatment,[15] and additionally, they were less likely than White patients to have a primary care provider.[16] These disparities highlight potential racial biases that can affect treatment decisions.

Access to Health Care

Health disparities related to access to health care manifest in various ways, particularly through barriers that prevent individuals from seeing a doctor.

---

[4] Ndugga, Pillai, and Artiga, "Disparities in Health."
[5] Institute of Medicine, *Racial and Ethnic Disparities*.   [6] Clair et al., "Disparities by Race."
[7] Schpero et al., "Blacks and Hispanics."
[8] Agency for Healthcare Research and Quality, *2023 National Healthcare Quality*.
[9] Best et al., "Racial Disparities."   [10] Hoffman et al., "Racial Bias."
[11] Sutton et al., "Racial and Ethnic Disparities."
[12] Institute of Medicine, *Racial and Ethnic Disparities*.
[13] Briesacher et al., "Racial and Ethnic Disparities."   [14] Barnett et al., "Racial Inequality."
[15] Parast et al., "Racial/Ethnic Differences."
[16] Centers for Disease Control and Prevention, *National Ambulatory Medical Care*.

One of the most critical barriers to accessing health care is the lack of insurance coverage. While the uninsured rate in the United States dropped by 18 percent during the pandemic,[17] approximately 26 million Americans remain uninsured, or about 8 percent of the US population, with a disproportionate number of those citizens being people of color.[18,19] Lacking health insurance can result in individuals delaying or forgoing necessary medical care due to the costs associated with doctor visits, dental care, medications, and treatments. Uninsured individuals are less likely to receive preventive care and necessary screenings, leading to late diagnoses of significantly worse health outcomes, including those for many types of cancer and cardiovascular risk factors.[20,21]

Health Care insurance aside, transportation and geographic constraints can likewise create barriers to accessing care. Transportation and geographic barriers significantly hinder access to health care services, especially for individuals in rural or underserved urban areas. Many patients struggle to reach health care facilities due to a lack of public transportation options or personal vehicle access. For example, about one in five individuals in low-income neighborhoods report transportation issues as their primary obstacle to seeing a doctor, with Black adults, families with low incomes, and adults with public health insurance being more likely to miss necessary care due to inadequate access to transportation.[22] As a result, patients can miss scheduled appointments or even avoid seeking care altogether, exacerbating health problems that could have otherwise been managed or prevented.

Broader Social Determinants of Health

Health disparities are further influenced by broader social determinants such as housing, food security, education, and employment. Housing instability is a major social determinant, with individuals experiencing housing instability being at a higher risk for conditions such as chronic diseases, mental health disorders, and poor self-rated health.[23] Specifically, the lack of stable housing can lead to increased stress, limited access to health care, and difficulties in medication adherence due to factors like

---

[17] National Center for Health Statistics, *U.S. Uninsured Rate Dropped*.
[18] Keisler-Starkey and Bunch, "Health Insurance Coverage."
[19] Hill, Artiga, and Damico, "Health Coverage by Race."
[20] Thomas et al., "Forgone Medical Care." [21] Ayanian et al., "Unmet Health Needs."
[22] Smith et al., "Transportation Barriers."
[23] Gu, Faulknerf, and Thorndike, "Housing Instability."

poor living conditions or overcrowding.[24] Individuals living in substandard housing often encounter barriers to accessing medical care, exacerbating health issues and the costs of care. **Food insecurity** is another key factor impacting health disparities, with households lacking stable access to sufficient food facing increased risks for various health conditions, including obesity, diabetes, and cardiovascular diseases.[25] Additionally, the stress and uncertainty surrounding food access can negatively impact mental health, contributing to anxiety and depression,[26] further highlighting how food security is integral to promoting overall health and well-being.

Other factors, such as education and employment, are critical to closing health disparity gaps. Adults with higher educational levels exhibit better health and reduced mortality rates compared to their less educated counterparts. Education influences health through several pathways, including improved health literacy, better job prospects, enhanced access to health care resources, and lower rates of unhealthy behaviors such as smoking and not engaging in physical activity.[27] Likewise, prolonged unemployment is associated with adverse physical and mental health outcomes, including increased rates of depression and chronic illness. Individuals in low-wage jobs often lack access to health insurance and face greater occupational hazards, exacerbating health risks. Providing stable, quality employment is therefore crucial for closing health disparity gaps and enhancing health outcomes, as consistent work can improve economic stability and social support systems.[28]

Addressing the SDOH is imperative to closing the persistent health equity gaps that plague the United States. By developing policy that is inclusive of these factors outside the US health care system, stakeholders can create targeted interventions that empower marginalized communities and ultimately lead to more equitable health outcomes. Investing in policies that improve living conditions, enhance access to nutritious foods, promote education and economic stability, and reduce systemic discrimination will forge pathways to better health for disadvantaged populations. Such a collective effort to address barriers rooted in the SDOH is not merely a goal; it is a necessity for achieving true health equity in the United States and ensuring that every individual has the opportunity to *live healthy lives*, regardless of their background or circumstances.

---

[24] Maqbool, Viveiros, and Ault, "Impacts of Affordable Housing."
[25] Beyene, "The Impact of Food Insecurity."
[26] Mousa, Remley, and Lane, "Food Systems, Food Insecurity."
[27] Zajacova and Lawrence, "Education and Health."   [28] Siegrist, "Health Inequalities."

8.2 The Principle of *Meeting People Where They Are*

Since Chapter 1, we've used the term *meeting people where they are*. We use this principle to emphasize the importance of understanding and addressing individuals' unique circumstances, needs, and contexts, rather than imposing a one-size-fits-all approach to health service delivery. This principle becomes especially relevant when considering how to close health disparities that persist in various communities across the United States. By adopting a patient-centered focus, health care providers can develop interventions that are tailored to the specific SDOH affecting different populations.

Meeting people where they are involves recognizing that patients come from diverse backgrounds and have unique experiences that may influence their access to health care and their health outcomes. This principle transcends mere physical location; it encompasses emotional and social contexts as well. For instance, patients may face barriers such as cultural or social mistrust of the health care system, or a lack of understanding regarding health information. Acknowledging such barriers is crucial to effectively engaging all communities in health care settings. As highlighted in the guidelines of Centers for Disease Control and Prevention, it is essential to learn the beliefs, attitudes, and values of the audience concerning health equity, to engage with them meaningfully.[29]

Meeting individuals where they are directly relates to enhancing health equity by addressing the root causes of health disparities. Health equity is grounded in the concept that everyone should have a fair and just opportunity to be as healthy as possible, which often requires tackling systemic and structural obstacles that disproportionately affect marginalized groups. By implementing strategies that reflect the realities of people's lives, such as providing services in community settings or engaging in culturally relevant communication, health care providers can alleviate some of these barriers. For example, organizations like Cityblock Health and the NIH Community Engagement Alliance have focused on closing health disparities by bringing care directly into communities, thereby establishing trust and relevance in their offerings.[30] These initiatives exemplify how this principle translates to practical actions that can lead to increased health service utilization and improved health outcomes among underserved populations.

Numerous community health initiatives have demonstrated the effectiveness of this principle. Mobile clinics, community health workers, and

---

[29] Centers for Disease Control and Prevention, *Communicating about Health Equity*.
[30] Zorthian, "'Meet People Where They Are.'"

outreach programs have been deployed to ensure that health care reaches patients where they live, work, and play – bringing services straight to underserved areas that typically struggle with access to traditional health care settings.[31] These programs often include screening for social drivers of health and connecting individuals to resources that extend beyond medical care, addressing issues such as housing, food insecurity, and transportation.[32]

The principle of *meeting people where they are* serves as a foundational aspect of addressing health disparities and promoting health equity. By tailoring health care delivery to meet individuals at their unique life circumstances, providers can overcome barriers that would otherwise prevent effective access to care. This approach not only enhances patient engagement but also fosters trust and community resilience. As the health care landscape continues to evolve, prioritizing this principle will be vital to creating a more equitable system that upholds the dignity of every individual and directly tackles the SDOH, impacting vulnerable populations.

8.3 Policy Considerations for Closing Health Disparity Gaps

In the United States, the health care debate tends to focus mostly on insurance for all. While access to health insurance is a critical part of any policy efforts to close health disparity gaps, this chapter highlights the need to go further. That said, in this section, we make considerations for inclusive health care policy that promotes equity not only for *seeing a doctor* (insurance for all) but also for *living healthy lives* (social determinants).

The Bloomberg Health Index ranks various countries based on their health care systems and overall health outcomes. Among the top twenty health care countries, a crucial aspect to examine is the availability of universal health care options. Universal health care is pivotal in ensuring that all citizens have access to essential health services without financial hardship. While the specific list may vary slightly, many of the countries generally recognized in the top tier of health care systems offer universal health care options. For example, countries like Spain, Italy, Iceland, Sweden, Australia, Singapore, and Norway are among the top-ranked in terms of health, and all have a robust universal health care system, or at the very least, a universal health care option that guarantees coverage for their entire populations. This commitment to universal coverage is linked to

---

[31] Baradaran, "Community Health Workers." [32] Baich, "Understanding Health Inequalities."

better health outcomes, lower health care costs, and increased overall life expectancy in these countries.[33]

Universal health care systems have garnered increasing attention as powerful frameworks for enhancing health outcomes across populations. By providing coverage to all individuals, regardless of socioeconomic status, these systems can ensure equitable access to essential health services, resulting in improved health care via the following metrics:

- *Improved access to care.* Countries with universal health care have notably lower rates of unmet health needs compared to those without comprehensive coverage.[34]
- *Enhanced preventative care.* The utilization of preventive health care services can allow for early disease detection and improved management, thereby reducing the progression of disease and curbing overall costs of care.[35]
- *Reduced health disparities.* Equitable health access ensures that all segments of the population, especially the most disadvantaged, receive the health care they need and enhances the holistic health of communities.[36]
- *Strengthened cost efficiency.* Access to an integrated, universal health care system would be economically efficient, with estimates that it would save over $450 billion per year if implemented in the United States.[37]

Globally, it is evident that universal health care plays an instrumental role in closing health disparity gaps through several interlinked mechanisms. Moreover, universal health care promotes equity and fosters a healthier overall population, reaffirming the critical role of comprehensive health coverage in public health strategy. Furthermore, it is critical that key policy considerations for closing health disparity gaps also address the SDOH as part of a holistic approach for identifying actionable strategies that can optimize health outcomes for all communities.

8.4 Strategies for Health Policy Change

Strategies for real change are uniquely challenging in the United States, in part due to stark party-line differences creating disagreement about how best to solve the problem of health care. The party-line differences must be considered when implementing any realistic, long-term

---

[33] Immad, "Countries with the Best Healthcare." [34] Wu et al., "Unmet Healthcare Needs."
[35] Wang and Lo, "Utilization of Preventive Care."
[36] Jindal et al., "Eliminating Healthcare Inequalities." [37] Blair, "335,000 Lives."

solutions to health care policy in the United States. From this perspective, bipartisan solutions must find a middle ground to drive policy solutions that are patient-centric but appeal to policy makers on both sides of the political aisle. In this section, we provide a framework for moving toward bipartisan solutions. Bipartisan policy is necessary to achieve long-term solutions that can endure from one election to another. For this reason, we focus on strategies that can coordinate across party lines.

Party-Line Differences in US Health Care Policy

In US politics, the left (Democratic Party) and the right (Republican Party) broadly differ on how they view the role of government. At a 10,000-foot overview, the left leans toward more government oversight in policy, with an emphasis on government regulation and accountability. The further right we go on the political spectrum, the less government oversight is favored in policy, with a greater emphasis on free-market competition and consumer choice. Generally speaking, the left sees the role of government as a critical part of policy solutions, and the right sees government as critical too, but only insofar as it is necessary to "keep the lights on" (i.e., its involvement should be limited to only those sectors where government is absolutely needed, like national defense). This broad contrast in perspective helps to explain, in part, their different positions on health care policy. To illustrate party-line differences in health care policy, Figure 8.2 outlines six key policy differences between the ACA (a Democrat-led legislation) and the American Health Care Act (AHCA; a Republican-led legislation).

Republicans generally advocate for a market-oriented approach to health care, believing that competition among private insurance providers leads to services of better quality and lower cost. Central to their perspective is the idea that individuals should have greater control and responsibility over their health care decisions. They often push for deregulation of the health care sector, arguing that reduced governmental oversight can spur innovation and efficiency.[38] For example, many Republicans support the repeal of the ACA, which they argue imposes burdensome mandates and costs on both health providers and consumers, suggesting that such an overreliance on government bureaucracy undermines personal choice and increases costs. Instead, Republicans often promote the use of Health Savings Accounts and tax credits to empower individuals to choose their

---

[38] The White House, *Congressional Republican Agenda*.

8.4 Strategies for Health Policy Change

Left (Democrat) ←		→ Right (Republican)
More federal government oversight in policy		Less federal government oversight in policy
Affordable Care Act (ACA; Obamacare)	**Policy**	**American Health Care Act (AHCA: Trumpcare)**
Required. All eligible citizens required to carry health insurance or pay a tax mandate.	Individual mandate	None. Continuous coverage is required with a 30% cost increase per month for failure to keep coverage.
All insurance policies required to carry coverage for ten essential health benefits.*	Essential health benefits	States decide whether to carry coverage for ten essential health benefits.
People with preexisting conditions cannot be denied coverage or charged higher rates.	Preexisting conditions	States decide whether insurers can charge more for people with preexisting conditions.
Optional, but would require high-deductible health plans and significant funding.	Health saving accounts	Tax-advantaged medical savings accounts for people to use as needed.
Expansion of Medicaid funding, meaning more people qualify.	Medicaid funding	Roll back Medicaid funding, meaning fewer people qualify.
People can deduct medical expenses only if costs exceed 10% of household adjusted gross income	Tax deductions	People can deduct the full cost of health insurance premiums from their annual federal tax returns
Achieved largely through enhanced federal regulation and oversight to gain accountability for pricing, and value-based reimbursement.	Party-line differences in health care delivery and for managing costs	Achieved largely through tax credits/deductions; empowering consumer choice; and greater market competition (nationally and internationally).

Figure 8.2 Six key policy differences between the ACA and the AHCA

insurance plans while simultaneously stressing the significance of reducing the overall cost of care through market-driven solutions. Their platforms frequently include proposals like block granting Medicaid to states, which allows for tailored approaches but also risks lowering standards of care for beneficiaries who rely on this program.[39]

[39] Physicians for a National Health Program, "Republican and Democratic Platforms."

Conversely, the Democratic Party approaches health care as a fundamental right, advocating for broader government involvement to ensure universal access to health care services. Democrats support expanding Medicare and Medicaid, for example, emphasizing that governmental intervention is necessary to protect vulnerable populations and bridge the gaps that are created by the private insurance market. Expectedly, the ACA, championed by Democrats, represents their commitment to increasing coverage and ensuring protections for patients with preexisting conditions. Democrats frequently promote a public option as a way to enhance competition and lower prices within the health care market, framing it as a step toward achieving universal coverage without mandating a complete overhaul of the existing system. Unlike their Republican counterparts, they argue that government negotiation of drug prices and health care costs can lead to significant savings for consumers and taxpayers alike, citing that such actions can reduce the overall financial burden of health care.[40]

Strategies for Change: Aligning Bipartisan Solutions

With a backdrop of ongoing discussions about health care inequities and access in the United States, bipartisan policy solutions that align public- and private-sector efforts are essential, as emphasized in Chapter 4. Bipartisan solutions should focus on developing partnerships that enhance health care delivery and address long-standing issues of health equity. The strategic alignment and collaboration between these sectors can lead to comprehensive initiatives that improve access to health care and ensure equitable treatment for underserved populations. Let us consider key areas where bipartisan support is most aligned.[41]

Expanding public–private partnerships (PPPs). PPPs can serve as a robust framework for enhancing health care access to address disparities. A significant area for improvement lies in the expansion of PPPs to leverage the strengths of both sectors. These partnerships can facilitate the sharing of resources, knowledge, and personnel, resulting in improved services delivered to historically marginalized communities. For example, developing initiatives that create a more integrated system of care can be achieved through partnerships that allow for the pooling of financial and technical resources for public health projects. Governments can also incentivize private-sector participation by providing grants or tax breaks aimed at

---

[40] Democratic National Committee, "Quality Healthcare."
[41] Bipartisan Policy Center, "Future of Healthcare."

improving health infrastructure in underserved areas. Such initiatives could direct the focus toward chronic disease management programs, preventive care, and wellness initiatives, catalyzing growth and responsiveness in health care delivery.

Enhancing telehealth services. In the wake of the COVID-19 pandemic, telehealth has emerged as a vital tool for enhancing access to health care services. Bipartisan efforts can be made to create policies that expand telehealth infrastructure, especially in rural and underserved urban areas where access to health care is limited. Policy makers should consider funding initiatives that encourage private companies to develop telehealth technologies tailored to the needs of diverse communities. For example, bipartisan legislation could support reimbursement for telehealth services across various insurance plans, which would ensure that health care providers are compensated adequately for virtual appointments. This could lead to increased provider participation in telehealth programs, ultimately enhancing patient access to care.

Addressing the 340B Drug Pricing Program. The 340B Drug Pricing Program, which mandates that drug manufacturers provide discounts on medications to eligible health care providers serving low-income patients, presents another area for potential bipartisan reform.[42] Policy makers can work collaboratively to ensure that this program is not only preserved but also enhanced to increase its effectiveness in addressing medication access for vulnerable populations. Enhancements could include stricter regulations regarding how savings from the program are utilized. Providers could be mandated to reinvest a percentage of savings back into community health initiatives, including preventive care and patient education programs, thereby promoting health equity.

Improving insurance coverage mechanisms. A critical bipartisan approach could focus on expanding insurance coverage mechanisms, particularly through Medicaid expansion in states that have yet to adopt it. This initiative can significantly reduce the number of uninsured individuals and provide low-income families with essential health care services. Additionally, the introduction of market reforms that enhance competition and transparency among insurance providers can help lower costs and improve access. Policies such as subsidies for low-income individuals to purchase health insurance on the exchanges can also promote greater insurance uptake. Such measures can be coupled with targeted outreach programs that educate and assist potential beneficiaries about available plans.

---

[42] Daly, "Bipartisan Healthcare Policy Changes."

Strengthening community health centers (CHCs). Investing in CHCs represents a major bipartisan health care solution. These centers play a crucial role by providing comprehensive services in underserved regions. Strengthening the funding for CHCs ensures their sustainability and their capacity to serve populations lacking access to primary care. Policies promoting the establishment of new CHCs in areas with demonstrated health care shortages would align public interests with private-sector investment in health. Furthermore, PPPs aimed at increasing the workforce within these centers can enhance their reach and efficacy. Incentives such as loan forgiveness and competitive salaries for professionals working in CHCs could attract more talented people to these critical areas of health care.

Addressing health care access and equity gaps in the United States necessitates a comprehensive range of bipartisan policy solutions. In Chapter 4, we outlined bipartisan solutions that can strengthen participation in health care by both the public and private sectors to make progress toward achieving universal health care. We started with the presumption that the United States is and will remain a mixed system in order to identify bipartisan solutions toward patient-centric health care policy. Collective public- and private-sector participation can enhance access to care (through universal coverage at a federal level) and close health equity gaps via the efficiencies of the private sector, which can include large socially oriented nonprofit organizations (e.g., donor-funded institutions and faith-based providers), and for-profit companies specifically tailored toward health care services, particularly in underserved communities (e.g., healthy food delivery companies with supply chain efficiencies to reach communities in "food deserts"). Ultimately, bipartisan support can bridge existing disparities and create holistic, sustainable frameworks for ongoing health care reform, ensuring that every American has access to quality health care they can afford.

It is also important to be considerate of long-term sustainability.[43] Short-term interventions, such as emergency funding or immediate health care programs, can offer critical support during crises, such as a pandemic or natural disaster. However, these interventions may fail to address the underlying structural issues that contribute to health disparities and inadequate health care access. Without a long-term strategy, the benefits of these short-term solutions may dissipate over time, leading to a cycle of recurring health crises and dependency on temporary fixes. Long-term

---

[43] Lennox et al., "Sustainability Approaches in Healthcare."

sustainability in health care policy ensures that resources are allocated efficiently, addresses the root causes of health inequities, and fosters resilience within health care systems. Sustainable practices in health care can lead to improvements in population health and more equitable access to care, ultimately reducing health care costs in the long run. By emphasizing the importance of balancing short-term interventions with long-term sustainability, policy makers can create a health care system that is not only responsive to immediate needs but also adaptive to future challenges.

8.5 Across the Pond: Addressing Social Determinants of Health

The significance of SDOH has been a focus in this chapter, and encompasses the lived environments where people are born, live, learn, work, play, worship, and age. In this section, we briefly explore the integration of policies related to housing and education within health care in Sweden and Denmark (two countries that have universal health care for all citizens), assessing their effectiveness compared to US policies. Countries like Sweden and Denmark have adopted comprehensive strategies that integrate policies addressing social determinants into their health care systems, fostering a holistic approach to health that emphasizes prevention and equitable access. In contrast, the United States often addresses health care in isolation, with a greater focus on the point of care than on the underlying social determinants that influence health outcomes.

In Sweden, public housing initiatives and supportive housing, combined with health care services, are integrated. The Danish model includes welfare provisions that offer housing support, including "Housing First" initiatives to provide stable housing as a platform for individuals experiencing homelessness, which is complemented by health services to enhance overall well-being. Such supportive housing policies not only reduce health care expenditures for high-cost users but also improve health outcomes significantly by facilitating access to necessary health services.[44] Conversely, housing interventions in the United States often occur independently from health care services, hindering their potential impact on public health. Although programs exist, such as supportive housing initiatives for low-income individuals, access to these services remains limited due to insufficient funding and bureaucratic hurdles. As a result, a significant number of eligible households do not receive federal rental assistance, leading to exacerbated health issues linked to housing instability.[45]

---

[44] Housing First Europe, "Denmark."   [45] Bailey, "Housing and Health Partners."

Now we turn to another key social determinant – education – Sweden and Denmark have integrative policies combining educational support with health services. In Sweden, for example, the integration of educational policies into health strategies is proactive. Schools not only provide education but also play a vital role in health promotion activities, including physical health, nutrition, and mental wellness programs. Denmark invests in education as a key determinant of health, with initiatives aimed at promoting health and well-being among school-aged children. The Danish health care system prioritizes health education in schools, significantly reducing the incidence of childhood obesity and mental health issues through early intervention programs.[46] In contrast, the US education system struggles with significant disparities in access to quality education, particularly in low-income and underserved communities. Although there are federally funded programs aimed at bridging these gaps, the efforts are often fragmented and under-resourced, limiting their effectiveness, and leaving children in these communities to face higher risks of health issues related to inadequate education and resources.[47]

The integration of policies addressing SDOH is crucial for establishing equitable health care systems. Countries like Sweden and Denmark exemplify successful frameworks that incorporate housing and education into their health care strategies, resulting in improved health outcomes and reduced disparities. In contrast, the US often treats these determinants separately, limiting the effectiveness of health interventions and perpetuating inequalities. By learning from the comprehensive approaches taken by other countries, such as by Scandinavian nations, the United States can enhance its health care system, ultimately leading to a healthier, more equitable society. The promotion of a health-in-all-policies framework that emphasizes the interconnectedness of the SDOH is essential for advancing population health and equity on a broader scale.

Chapter Summary

Achieving health equity is not only a moral imperative, but it is also a feasible goal if policies are designed to address both access to health care and the broader SDOH. Health equity requires a comprehensive approach that considers systemic inequities, access barriers, and the environmental, social, and economic factors shaping health outcomes. Policies

---

[46] European Commission, *Health and Well-Being*.
[47] Levinson, Geller, and Allen, "Social Determinants of Learning."

such as universal health care systems, Medicaid expansion, and community health initiatives provide valuable examples of how addressing these barriers can bridge the gaps in access and outcomes. Efforts like the ACA and the NHS demonstrate that, while challenging, systemic change is possible with intentional policy design.

By meeting people where they are and tailoring interventions to address diverse needs, policy makers can foster a more inclusive health care system. Integrating SDOH into health care policy is essential for reducing disparities and promoting well-being across all population segments. This holistic approach not only enhances access to care but also addresses the root causes of health inequities. Achieving health equity will require sustained investment, bipartisan collaboration, and a commitment to tackling long-standing disparities. While challenges remain, the pathway to health equity is clear: creating a system where every individual has a fair opportunity to live a healthy life, regardless of their circumstances. Through innovative, inclusive, and data-driven strategies, health equity is not just a possibility – it is an achievable reality.

CHAPTER 9

Moving toward More Inclusive Health Care Policy

Insights

- Policies must address financial, geographic, linguistic, and cultural barriers to ensure equitable and accessible health care for all individuals.
- Inclusive policies consider clinical needs, financial realities, and lifestyle factors for holistic health care solutions.
- Training providers in empathy and cultural competence fosters trust, enhances communication, and improves health outcomes for diverse populations.
- Cross-sector partnerships addressing SDOH, like housing and education, are vital for reducing health disparities and improving outcomes.
- Countries like Germany and Sweden demonstrate integrated systems aligning health care with social determinants for better patient engagement and equity.

Health disparities are persistent challenges that reflect underlying social and economic inequities. From chronic disease conditions, such as diabetes and hypertension, to uninsurance rates, and barriers to care that extend beyond mere access – such as affordability, quality of care received, and treatment – health disparities can vary substantially by race and socioeconomic status.[1] The pursuit of an inclusive health care policy in the United States has become increasingly crucial as disparities in health outcomes continue to persist among different demographic groups. Moving toward a more inclusive health care policy is multifaceted to ensure that policy and social determinants of health (SDOH) are integrated. It requires a collaborative approach that expands access to care, addresses the SDOH, promotes cultural competence, and implements equitable policies. By adapting policies to the needs of underserved communities and

[1] Ndugga, Pillai, and Artiga, "Disparities in Health."

systematically addressing the barriers they face, any nation can make significant strides toward improving the overall health and well-being of *all* its citizens.

At its core, **inclusive health care** is a system of health care that thoroughly integrates principles of equity and accessibility at all levels of health care delivery. This integration means policies are designed to provide health services *and* ensure that these services are accessible, acceptable, and of high quality for every individual in a population, including marginalized, underserved, and vulnerable groups.[2] Inclusive policies aim to eliminate or overcome barriers – whether they are financial, geographic, linguistic, or cultural – allowing all individuals to obtain the care that is not only necessary but also appropriate to their specific context and needs. In this way, an inclusive policy framework can lead to more than just collective health benefits; it can transform the relationship between communities and health care providers by fostering communication and trust through culturally competent care, thereby empowering patients to take active roles in managing their health, which leads to higher patient satisfaction, improved adherence to treatment plans, and, ultimately, better health outcomes.[3] In short, inclusive health care is considerate of the barriers that prevent people not only from *seeing a doctor* (insurance for all) but also from *living healthy lives* (social determinants).

9.1 The Whole Being Model: A Holistic Approach

In this chapter, we take a unique approach to discussing inclusive care by using the **whole being model** framework[4] to connect with the discussion of how to move toward a more inclusive health care policy. Using this model as a framework in health care, the *whole being* is reflected by the patient, the consumer, and the person. Using this framework, which humanizes individuals as being more than just *patients* within the health care ecosystem, Figure 9.1 illustrates each component of the whole being and shows how it is connected to fourteen key steps that are necessary to move toward a more inclusive health care policy in the United States.

The whole being model, articulated by the authors of this text in their work *Patient-Centric Analytics in Health Care*, serves as a framework for understanding patient care through the lens of the drivers for the health

---

[2] Special Olympics Health, "Inclusive Health."
[3] Health Research & Educational Trust, "Culturally Competent Healthcare."
[4] Gillespie and Privitera, *Patient-Centric Analytics*.

Ensure Health Care Workforce Diversity: Encourage diversity in the health care workforce to reflect the populations being served.

Expand Health Care Coverage: Ensure universal health coverage by adopting policies that provide affordable health care access to all individuals.

Improve Access to Mental Health Services: Expand mental health care access, particularly for marginalized communities, and integrate mental health services into primary care.

Strengthen Community Health Resources: Invest in community health centers and mobile clinics to provide care to underserved and rural populations.

Implement Patient-Centered Care Models: Focus on care models that prioritize the individual needs and preferences of diverse patient groups.

Promote Health Literacy: Develop programs to improve health literacy, empowering individuals to understand and navigate health care systems.

Foster Collaboration Across Sectors: Engage stakeholders from public sectors, private sectors, and communities to develop comprehensive, inclusive health policies.

Advocate for Equity-Focused Legislation: Support and enact laws that eliminate discrimination and bias in health care systems and policies.

Utilize Technology and Telehealth: Expand telehealth services to improve access for remote and underserved populations while ensuring digital equity.

Incorporate LGBTQ+-Inclusive Policies: Establish policies and training to address the unique health care needs of LGBTQ+ individuals.

Support Aging Populations: Expand resources and care options for older adults, including culturally sensitive geriatric care.

Address Health Care Inequities: Develop initiatives to reduce disparities in health outcomes based on race, ethnicity, gender, disability, geography, and socioeconomic status.

Promote Cultural Competency: Train care providers in cultural competence to promote understanding and improve communication with diverse populations.

Integrate Social Determinants of Health: Incorporate strategies to address factors such as housing, education, nutrition, and transportation that affect health outcomes.

Consumer

Patient

Person

Whole Being

Figure 9.1 The whole being model in health care: patient, person, and consumer – connected to fourteen key steps needed in the United States to move toward a more inclusive health care policy

Source: Gillespie and Privitera (2018)

9.1 The Whole Being Model: A Holistic Approach

care decisions that people make. This model emphasizes the integration of various dimensions of how decisions are made by the *people being served* (i.e., those who we typically refer to as patients) in health care settings. The *whole being* of an individual consists of three dimensions or roles:

- *Patient.* The patient is who we are at the point of care. The drivers of health care decisions of the patient include care incentives, maximizing comfort, and minimizing pain, suffering, morbidity, and mortality.
- *Consumer.* The consumer is considerate of how much care costs. The drivers of health care decisions of the consumer include financial incentives, minimizing costs, and maximizing value.
- *Person.* The person encompasses who we are and how we live. The drivers of health care decisions of the person include social and cultural incentives, minimizing daily inconvenience, and maximizing lifestyle.

Using this framework, the individual operates in three distinct but interrelated roles: the patient, who seeks medical treatment and care; the consumer, who navigates the market aspects of health services, including costs and access; and the person, whose life choices and behaviors impact overall health. The interplay between these roles can sometimes lead to conflict. Consider a scenario where the cost of a lifesaving medication places a financial burden on the consumer aspect of an individual, while the patient role advocates for access to that treatment. Such conflicts underscore the necessity of inclusive health care policies that address the diverse needs and challenges faced by individuals.

Inclusive health care policy must recognize and mitigate the friction between these roles to enhance patient experiences and outcomes. Using the whole being model, policy makers can attentively develop strategies that encompass not only clinical needs but also the financial realities that individuals face as consumers and the behavioral choices they make as persons. For example, when policy frameworks integrate affordability measures for medications, they ease the financial burden on patients while still prioritizing health outcomes. This represents a balancing act that can lead to a reduction in health disparities stemming from socioeconomic inequities. Likewise, if incentives were provided to the patient for achieving health outcomes, this could drive changes in their behaviors as a person and potentially bolster their ability to reach health goals.

This framework also lends itself to leveraging analytics in decision-making. Analytics can help identify patients who may struggle with their roles or face barriers based on their individual circumstances, thus facilitating tailored interventions. For example, policies that encourage the use of health apps or telemedicine can empower patients to take charge of their health management while also addressing consumer interests through accessible and cost-effective solutions. This dual emphasis on consumer engagement alongside patient care underlines the shifting responsibilities among stakeholders in the health care ecosystem. The model thus promotes a collaborative environment in which patients receive holistic support, leading to better adherence to preventive measures and health management practices.

A substantive shift, brought about by the whole being model, is the move toward shared responsibility among providers and payers in addressing both patient and consumer needs. In traditional health care settings, these roles were often siloed, leading to increased tension between physicians and insurers. The model proposes an integrated approach where both parties collaborate to create a more seamless experience for patients, ultimately supporting inclusive decision-making. By aligning incentives for providers with the financial capabilities of consumers, health care policies can promote practices aimed at early detection and prevention, ultimately resulting in cost savings for both individuals and the health care system. This holistic approach advocates for policies that align the goals of individual health outcomes with broader societal health objectives, demonstrating a commitment to addressing the needs of all roles encompassed by the *whole being*. The principles articulated with this framework stand as foundational elements for reforming health care policies that truly reflect the diverse needs of individuals in society.

9.2 Steps toward Inclusive Health Care Policy

Moving toward a more inclusive health care policy in the United States will certainly require collaboration across federal, state, and local governments, private institutions, and community organizations. As discussed in Chapter 8, promoting an inclusive health care system will also require collaborative, bipartisan work in developing policy that puts the *whole being* at the center of the health care model. In Figure 9.1, fourteen key steps toward a more inclusive policy are identified. In the figure, note that the steps are organized across the three dimensions or roles of the whole being in a way that aligns closely to their interests. In the next section, we briefly look at each step (from bottom left to right in Figure 9.1) and provide an example to elucidate the tangible actions that are being taken toward more inclusive health care.

Advocate for equity-focused legislation. Equity-focused legislation refers to laws aimed at dismantling barriers that result in inequitable health care delivery. These laws are designed to ensure that marginalized populations receive fair and equitable treatment in health services. Such legislation typically encompasses antidiscrimination provisions that specifically address race, ethnicity, gender identity, disability, and other protected statuses. Section 1557 in the Affordable Care Act (ACA) is one example of equity-focused legislation in that it prohibits discrimination based on race, color, national origin, sex, age, or disability in health programs receiving federal financial assistance.[5] By proactively addressing disparities through legislative means, health care systems can achieve equitable health care for all populations.

Promote health literacy. Health literacy entails more than just reading and interpreting medical information; it encompasses the capacities to understand health-related concepts, communicate health needs, and navigate complex health systems. Individuals with adequate health literacy are better equipped to understand medical instructions, engage in preventive health behaviors, and manage chronic conditions effectively.[6] The **Health Literacy Action Plan** of the Centers for Disease Control and Prevention exemplifies a strategic approach to promote health literacy as part of inclusive health policy. The plan outlines specific goals and strategies aimed at improving health literacy across diverse groups. It recognizes that many individuals struggle to access and comprehend health information due to various SDOH, including education level, language proficiency, and cultural barriers.[7]

Implement patient-centered care models. Patient-centered care emphasizes the importance of understanding each patient's experience, values, and circumstances while involving them as partners in their own health care decisions. This approach is vital for addressing health disparities and ensuring equitable health access for all populations. The **Patient-Centered Medical Home (PCMH)** model exemplifies how patient-centered care can be effectively implemented within an inclusive health care framework.[8] Originally developed in the 1960s but gaining substantial traction in the 2000s, PCMH is designed to provide continuous, coordinated care that is responsive to patients' individual needs and preferences. The PCMH model operates on key principles that align closely with

---

[5] 116th Congress, *Equal Healthcare*.   [6] Fleary and Ettienne, "Social Disparities in Health Literacy."
[7] U.S. Centers for Disease Control and Prevention, *Health Literacy Action Plan*.
[8] U.S. Centers for Disease Control and Prevention, *Patient-Centered Medical Home*.

inclusive health care policy goals: (i) comprehensive care, including both mental health and social determinants, and ensuring holistic and coordinated care across provider settings, (ii) patient engagement and empowerment encouraging patients to actively participate in their own care planning and decision-making processes, (iii) improved access to health care services through extended hours, telehealth options, and proactive communication strategies, (iv) team-based care fostering collaborative care teams consisting of various health professionals working together to support patient needs, and (v) quality and safety monitoring with providers routinely assessing patient outcomes and satisfaction, allowing them to adapt their practices to better serve the communities where they operate.

Strengthen community health resources. Community health centers (CHCs) and mobile clinics are instrumental in overcoming barriers related to location, economic status, and systemic inequities in health care systems. These resources function as safety nets, delivering care to individuals and communities who might otherwise face significant obstacles to accessing health services. Investments in CHCs and mobile clinics increase health care access by providing services where they are needed the most. Their approach is proactive, offering a wide range of medical, dental, and mental health services tailored to the specific needs of the communities they serve. The **Health Center Program** in the United States epitomizes a successful approach to strengthening community health resources and exemplifies the integration of inclusive health care policy.[9] Established under the Public Health Service Act in 1965, this program has evolved into a national network of CHCs that provide comprehensive and affordable care, irrespective of patients' ability to pay. Similar to the PCMH model, CHCs operate on key principles that align closely with inclusive health care policy goals by being adaptive in their practices to better serve diverse populations.

Improve access to mental health services. Mental health is an integral aspect of overall health, and access to mental health services must be equitable and inclusive to ensure that all individuals receive the support they need. As primary care settings are typically the first point of contact for individuals seeking health care, they represent an ideal location for providing mental health services. By embedding mental health care within primary care, we can reduce stigma, enhance care coordination, and promote holistic health management. The **Mental Health Parity and Addiction Equity Act**, a groundbreaking piece of legislation in 2008, provides an exemplar for

---

[9] Health Resources & Services Administration, "Health Center Program."

improving access to mental health services in the United States. This act, most recently updated in September 2024, ensures that individuals who have group health plans or individual health insurance and who seek treatment for covered *mental health or substance-use disorders* do not face greater burdens to access benefits for those conditions or disorders than they would face when seeking coverage for the treatment of a medical condition or a surgical procedure.[10] Moving forward, it is essential to continue examining additional strategies to promote mental health care access, ensuring that all individuals can receive the comprehensive care they seek.

Expand health care coverage. While the ACA was implemented to bring a universal health care option to Americans, its rollout has been greatly interrupted due, in large part, to an inability to gain bipartisan support for the policy. Universal health coverage, however, is critical not only for the promotion of public health but also for enhancing health equity in society. Among the top thirty countries in the Bloomberg Global Health Index 2024 rankings, several have established universal health care or options. Spain, Italy, and Sweden, for example, have robust public-health systems that ensure coverage for all residents. Countries that implement universal health care often report lower rates of preventable deaths and higher overall life expectancies compared to those lacking such systems.[11] The **Children's Health Insurance Program (CHIP)** serves as an excellent example of a US policy that has successfully expanded health care coverage to ensure affordable access for children in lower-income families. Established in 1997, CHIP was designed to provide health insurance to uninsured children from families that earn too much money to qualify for Medicaid but not enough to afford private coverage.[12] Expanding such universal coverage to all Americans is a critical step toward meeting people where they are, in order to ensure equitable access to affordable, quality health care.

Ensure health care workforce diversity. Ensuring health care workforce diversity is an essential component of inclusive health care policy, aimed at creating a workforce that reflects the diversity of the populations it serves. By embracing diversity in health care professions, the system can foster more culturally competent care, which ultimately leads to improved communication with patients, greater comfort and trust with providers, more tailored care plans, and better health outcomes for all individuals.[13] In the

---

[10] U.S. Centers for Medicare & Medicaid Services, *Mental Health Parity*.
[11] World Population Review, "Healthiest Countries 2024."
[12] HealthCare.gov, *Children's Health Insurance Program*.
[13] Coronado et al., "Dynamics of Diversity."

United States, the **National Health Service Corps (NHSC)**, established in 1970, is a notable example of a policy designed to promote health care workforce diversity by incentivizing health professionals to practice in underserved communities through scholarships, recruitment, community engagement, and training. The NHSC aims to improve access to primary health care in areas experiencing shortages of health care providers, particularly in rural and low-income urban areas.[14] Prioritizing workforce diversity will remain essential for fostering a responsive health care system that meets the needs of all individuals within the community.

Foster collaboration across sectors. In health care, many determinants of health – such as socioeconomic status, education, and environment – extend beyond the traditional boundaries of health care services. Effective health policies must consider these diverse factors by engaging various stakeholders, including health care providers, community organizations, government agencies, and private-sector partners. Collaboration across sectors fosters a comprehensive understanding of the community's needs, enabling policy makers to develop inclusive health interventions that address health disparities tailored to each community. The **Accountable Health Communities model** is a pioneering US policy initiative launched by the Centers for Medicare & Medicaid Services (CMS) to improve health outcomes for Medicare and Medicaid beneficiaries by identifying and addressing nonmedical factors that influence health. Key benefits of cross-sector collaboration include: (i) holistic solutions via coordinated efforts between health care, education, housing, and employment sectors, (ii) resource allocation by pooling of resources, knowledge, and expertise across sectors, and (iii) community engagement and empowerment.[15] Emphasizing cross-sector collaboration is essential to give communities a voice in their health care needs that can lead to creating policies that holistically support the health and well-being of all individuals and communities.

Utilize technology and telehealth. The COVID-19 pandemic has accelerated the adoption of **telehealth** services, revealing technology's potential to bridge the gaps in access to care and improve health outcomes for individuals facing challenges such as geographic isolation, transportation barriers, and limited health care resources. Utilizing technology and telehealth is therefore essential for creating inclusive health care policies that improve access for remote and underserved populations. **Federally Qualified**

---

[14] National Health Service Corps, *Mission, Work, and Impact.*
[15] U.S. Centers for Medicare & Medicaid Services, *Accountable Health Communities Model.*

9.2 Steps toward Inclusive Health Care Policy

Health Centers (FQHCs) are community-based nonprofit health care centers that receive federal funding to deliver primary care services including telehealth services and community outreach to underserved populations in the United States.[16] FQHCs serve as an example of how technology and telehealth initiatives can effectively improve access for remote and underserved populations. Telehealth has become a vital tool in health care delivery, allowing patients to access services remotely via digital platforms. This utilization of technology provides numerous benefits that contribute to inclusive health care policies, including: (i) increased access to care, (ii) enhanced continuity of care, (iii) convenience, and (iv) cost effectiveness.[17]

Incorporate LGBTQ+-inclusive policies. The unique health care needs of LGBTQ+ individuals stem from a lifetime of adversities, including stigma, discrimination, and inadequate cultural competency among providers. Such policies are vital to promoting an environment of inclusivity, enhancing health outcomes, and fostering trust between LGBTQ+ patients and health care providers. The **Human Rights Campaign's Health Care Equality Index (HEI)** serves as a powerful example of an initiative designed to promote LGBTQ+-inclusive policies within US health care organizations (HCOs). Established in 2007, the HEI provides a framework for health care facilities to assess their policies and practices concerning LGBTQ+ patient care. Key features of this framework include: (i) setting standards of care, (ii) providing training and resources, (iii) evaluation and accountability, (iv) recognition for those facilities that meet or exceed standards, and (v) community engagement.[18] By establishing and promoting such inclusive initiatives, health care providers and physicians can create a welcoming environment where LGBTQ+ individuals receive culturally competent, equitable care.

Support aging populations. As populations across the world age, the need for inclusive health care policies that support older adults has become increasingly critical. With one in five adults expected to be aged sixty-five or older in the United States by 2030, and with those adults being more racially diverse and in need of more focused care (e.g., chronic disease is more prevalent among older adults), the growing number of aging adults will create a greater demand for caregivers, including family members and professionals.[19] The combination of aging adults and shrinking younger

---
[16] HealthCare.gov, *Federally Qualified Health Center.*
[17] Anawade, Sharma, and Gahane, "Impact of Telemedicine."
[18] Human Rights Campaign Foundation, "Healthcare Equality Index 2024."
[19] United States Census Bureau, *Baby Boomers.*

population cohorts may even exacerbate labor shortages in the caregiving sector, impacting the delivery of services. Supporting aging populations through the expansion of resources and care options is therefore crucial for fostering inclusive health care policies. The **Older Americans Act**, enacted in 1965, serves as an exemplary model for expanding resources and care options that prioritize inclusivity and cultural sensitivity in geriatric care through: (i) programs and services, (ii) state and community grants, (iii) advocacy, (iv) culturally sensitive care, and (v) a focus on health and nutrition.[20] Investing in the well-being of older adults is not only a matter of social responsibility, but it is also essential to enhancing the overall health of our communities.

Address health care inequities. Health Care inequities encompass systemic and structural barriers that prevent specific populations from receiving access to high-quality health care. The significance of addressing these inequities is evident by: (i) disproportionate health outcomes, (ii) SDOH, (iii) legal and ethical considerations, (iv) economic impact, and (v) the diversity of patient needs. The ACA, enacted in 2010, represents a monumental US policy initiative aimed at reducing health care disparities in the United States through various provisions, including: (i) expanded coverage to ensure access to insurance for all Americans, (ii) provisions that prohibit discrimination such as Section 1557 in the ACA, (iii) focus on preventative and essential services, (iv) funding of CHCs, (v) the collection of health data to ensure culturally competent care, and (vi) health equity initiatives to close health equity gaps.[21] As the nation continues to confront challenges related to health care policy, leveraging greater bipartisan support for the ACA, or an iteration of it, will be crucial to meaningfully addressing health care inequities in the United States.

Promote cultural competency. Cultural competency in health care refers to the ability of providers to understand, respect, and effectively interact with patients from diverse cultural backgrounds. As the US population continues to grow more diverse, the importance of integrating cultural competency into health care policy has become increasingly significant. Training care providers in cultural competence is essential to improving understanding, enhancing communication, and ultimately delivering high-quality care to all individuals, regardless of their backgrounds. The US Department of Health and Human Services (HHS) recognizes the importance of cultural competency in health care by implementing various

---

[20] Administration for Community Living, *Older Americans Act*.
[21] 111th Congress, *Affordable Care Act*.

initiatives, such as the **HHS Cultural Competency Training initiative**, aimed at training providers to meet the needs of culturally diverse populations.[22] This initiative is comprehensive and includes a range of training programs, such as free online courses and a curriculum that is integrated into medical education settings. Prioritizing cultural competency can not only benefit patients but also strengthen the integrity and responsiveness of health care delivery.

Integrate SDOH. A theme throughout many of the steps described in this section is the emphasis on SDOH to achieve inclusive health care policy. Integrating strategies to address these determinants within health care policy is essential for creating a more inclusive health system that *meets people where they are* to promote equitable health outcomes across diverse populations. In the United States, the CMS has implemented initiatives to address SDOH among Medicaid and Medicare beneficiaries. For example, CMS has introduced new flexibilities to address SDOH through the provision of health-related social-needs services, such as housing support, nutritional assistance, and transportation services. Other services include "in-lieu-of" services, which allow CMS to cover nontraditional, preventive services that can improve health outcomes.[23] For example, if a patient faces housing instability, they can receive housing-related support as a substitute for more urgent medical care, thereby addressing the underlying social issue. By allowing flexibility in Medicaid programs, emphasizing collaboration with community organizations, and advocating for comprehensive data collection, CMS is leading the charge in creating a more equitable health care landscape.

The steps toward a more inclusive health care policy in the United States emphasize a holistic, collaborative approach that integrates diverse sectors, addresses health disparities, and focuses on the well-being of all individuals. Key strategies include advocating for equity-focused legislation, promoting health literacy, implementing patient-centered care models, and strengthening community health resources. Additionally, improving mental health access, expanding coverage, ensuring workforce diversity, and fostering cross-sector collaboration are crucial. Technology and telehealth, LGBTQ+-inclusive policies, support for aging populations, and addressing SDOH will further enhance inclusivity. By prioritizing these actions universally, the United States can move toward a health care system that is equitable, accessible, and responsive to the needs of diverse populations.

---

[22] U.S. Department of Health & Human Services, *Advancing Health Equity.*
[23] Medicaid.gov, *Health Related Social Needs.*

9.3 Closing Health Disparity Gaps: Key Themes

Addressing health disparities is a pressing need within the health care system, as these disparities can significantly affect population health, particularly among marginalized and underserved communities. The theme of closing health disparity gaps encompasses several critical elements, with a focus on the interplay between: (i) empathy and the etiology of health disparities, (ii) cultural diversity and diagnosis, and (iii) at a provider level, listening to patients more than simply hearing them.

Empathy + Etiology. Empathy plays an essential role in addressing health disparities. It allows health care providers to genuinely understand and connect with patients, enabling them to recognize the unique challenges faced by individuals from diverse backgrounds. When providers demonstrate empathy, they can create an environment that fosters trust and open communication, which is essential for effective treatment. Empathetic interactions can also improve patient adherence to treatment plans, enhance patient satisfaction, and ultimately result in better health outcomes. To embed empathy within health policy and practice, several strategies can be implemented, including: (i) developing training programs focused on cultural competency and empathy, (ii) adopting policies from HCOs that prioritize empathetic care, encouraging staff to engage with patients in a supportive and understanding manner, and (iii) evaluating the impact of these empathetic practices on patient outcomes to facilitate continuous improvement in health care delivery.

Culture + Diagnosis. The interplay between culture and diagnosis is crucial for closing health disparity gaps. By acknowledging the influence of cultural backgrounds on health perceptions and treatment, addressing biases within health care delivery, and implementing proactive policies for culturally competent care, HCOs can work toward achieving equitable access to quality care for all individuals. One of the key spaces where culture and diagnosis are most evident is at the point of care. Indeed, patients who share the same ethnic background as their physician report being more satisfied with their care, in part due to the trust they have for the care they receive.[24] In this way, HCOs can adopt policies that promote the recruitment of a diverse workforce, reflecting the communities they serve. By fostering an environment of trust and inclusivity, health care systems can strengthen patient–provider relationships and improve overall health outcomes.

---

[24] Takeshita et al., "Racial/Ethnic and Gender Concordance."

Listening > Hearing. The distinction between listening and merely hearing is crucial in health care interactions. Hearing refers to the physiological process of perceiving sounds, whereas listening involves actively engaging with and comprehending the speaker's message. Effective listening requires focus, empathy, and an understanding of the patient's context, which ultimately enhances patient engagement and care delivery. By prioritizing listening, health care providers can cultivate an environment that encourages open communication by demonstrating genuine interest and empathy toward patients. Techniques such as maintaining eye contact, asking open-ended questions, and providing feedback can help facilitate a productive dialogue. Additionally, training programs focused on developing active listening skills and practicing mindfulness can strengthen listening skills and equip health care professionals with the tools necessary to engage with patients effectively. When health care providers actively listen to their patients, it fosters a sense of trust, making patients feel valued and understood. This sense of trust can encourage patients to express their concerns more openly and to adhere to treatment recommendations.[25] Also, patients who feel heard are more likely to report higher levels of satisfaction with their care, leading to improved health outcomes and overall experiences in the health care system.[26] By understanding the difference between listening and hearing, adopting strategies to enhance active listening, and recognizing the positive impacts on trust and patient satisfaction, health care providers can better serve diverse populations.

9.4 Humanizing Patients in the Health Care Ecosystem

Recognizing that patients are more than just their illnesses is crucial for creating an empathetic health care approach. Health Care providers should focus on the holistic view of patients, acknowledging their individual experiences, emotions, and personal histories, rather than merely treating their symptoms or medical conditions. By fostering relationships that honor each patient's unique narrative, health care professionals can improve the overall care experience and outcomes.[27]

Bridging gaps between the perspectives of the patient, consumer, and person involves recognizing the distinct, yet interconnected, roles that patients play in the health care system. Effective communication and understanding among health care providers, patients, and payers are

---

[25] Authenticx, "Actively Listening."   [26] Worrall, "What Is Patient Experience."
[27] Busch et al., "Humanization of Care."

essential for creating a care model that addresses the concerns of all stakeholders. Integrating patient feedback into care delivery can facilitate a more collaborative environment where their needs and preferences are genuinely valued. Frameworks for creating human-centric health care environments include fostering emotional connections, ensuring patient dignity, and encouraging participation in care decisions. Implementing strategies that emphasize empathy and respect leads to improved patient–provider relationships, which, in turn, can enhance engagement and satisfaction.[28] By adopting holistic practices and training staff to prioritize patient-centered care, health care institutions can significantly enrich the overall patient experience.

Policy makers must consider diverse perspectives and the lived experiences of patients to create guidelines that reflect their needs. Incorporating patient perspectives into health policy decisions can lead to more effective and equitable health care solutions that recognize the complexities of individual circumstances. Programs that prioritize person-centered approaches, for example, have demonstrated improvements in patient satisfaction and engagement as well as reductions in hospital readmissions.[29] Such evidence can help persuade policy makers to integrate these successful strategies into broader health care policies.

To bring together each of the themes discussed in the last two sections, consider the following anecdote from an actual point-of-care experience of an expectant mother receiving a miscarriage diagnosis.

> On that day, she lay on an exam table, her hands clasped tightly over the slight curve of her belly, a small comfort in her husband's absence. Sixteen weeks. Today, she would hear her baby's heartbeat, maybe even learn the sex of her child.
>
> The doctor entered without preamble, his white coat swishing as he moved to the machine. He offered no greeting, barely glancing her way as he applied the icy gel to her stomach. She turned her head to the screen, her heart pounding with nervous excitement.
>
> Seconds passed. The doctor's hand stilled. His face betrayed nothing but a tightening of his jaw.
>
> "What's wrong?" she asked, her voice cracking under the weight of the unspoken answer.
>
> "There's no heartbeat," he said flatly, not looking at her.
>
> Her world tilted. "No . . . heartbeat?" she whispered, barely able to form the words.

---

[28] Merahn, "Humanizing Healthcare." [29] Marzban et al., "Impact of Patient Engagement."

"The baby is not alive," he continued, already pulling off his gloves. "A nurse will be in shortly to explain next steps." He turned, leaving the room without so much as a glance back.

The door clicked shut and the silence became unbearable. Her breath caught in her chest as tears blurred her vision. Alone in the sterile room, she clutched her belly, the joy she'd carried for sixteen weeks, replaced by a hollow ache – and a grief magnified by the cold, clinical detachment of the news.

In this example, the doctor provided a diagnosis – but without empathy, without consideration for her as a woman, and without truly listening to her responsiveness in reaction to the devastating diagnosis. She was left alone in mental anguish as the doctor left, satisfied that he technically did his job; he did not do his job at all. He failed her. At the point of care, applying these key themes into practice is fundamental to putting the *care* in the practice of *health care*.

9.5 Across the Pond: The Whole Being Model in Policy

In the United States, health care policies predominantly reflect a fragmented system where the roles of patient, consumer, and person are often misaligned. The ACA, particularly its Medicaid expansion provisions, made strides toward improving health care access for low-income populations. However, its implementation has been uneven across states, currently with ten states still not adopting the expansion.[30] This inconsistency has led to significant gaps in coverage and health services for vulnerable populations, effectively neglecting the person role that emphasizes individual experiences and needs.

Moreover, US health policies have traditionally prioritized cost-effectiveness over holistic care. For instance, while policies like the **Patients' Bill of Rights** promote informed patient choices, they largely focus on the transactional aspects of health care rather than fostering deeper engagement with patients as partners in care.[31] This framework often fails to encourage patients to participate actively in their health management, placing them in a passive role, primarily as consumers of medical services. In addition, the focus on consumerism in health – propelled by market-driven policies – further complicates the American health care landscape. The push for price transparency, while aimed at

---

[30] Kaiser Family Foundation, "Medicaid Expansion Decisions."
[31] U.S. Department of State, *Patient Bill of Rights*.

enhancing consumer choice, sometimes overlooks patients' needs for comprehensive care that transcend financial considerations. As a result, many patients feel unprepared to navigate the complexities of health care decision-making, limiting their ability to act as informed consumers.[32]

In contrast, several other nations have adopted more integrated approaches in their health care policies that explicitly address the patient, consumer, and person framework. For example, Germany operates on a social insurance model that emphasizes solidarity and inclusivity, which ensures that all citizens have access to comprehensive health coverage, regardless of their socioeconomic status.[33] Here, the roles of patient and person are more seamlessly interwoven, as health care services are designed to consider the holistic needs of individuals, including SDOH.

In nations like Canada and the Nordic countries, health systems are structured around universal coverage principles, aligning closely with the whole being model.[34,35] These systems inherently support the patient role by removing financial barriers to access, thereby facilitating health equity. Policies in these countries also promote preventive care and public health initiatives which recognize the importance of individual and community health beyond just medical treatment. Also, the integration of social services with health care in countries like Australia reflects a comprehensive understanding of individuals as whole beings. Programs that address housing, educational opportunities, and mental health are entrenched within their health care policies, acknowledging that health outcomes are deeply affected by varied life experiences and environmental contexts.[36]

The divergence in policies between the United States and other countries underscores crucial differences in how each system supports or neglects the patient, consumer, and person roles. The complexity of the US health care system often relegates patients to fragmented roles, emphasizing either illness management or consumer aspects, thereby sidestepping the broader view of individuals as whole beings who are navigating their own health journeys. On the contrary, countries with universal coverage and integrated services recognize the multifaceted needs of their populations and create policies that encourage meaningful patient engagement. Adopting the whole being model is therefore essential, allowing for

---

[32] Sinaiko, Bambury, and Chien, "Consumer Choice."
[33] Busse et al., "Health Insurance in Germany."
[34] Martin et al., "Canada's Universal Health-care System."
[35] Frelle-Petersen, Hein, and Christiansen, "Nordic Social Welfare Model."
[36] Davies et al., "Healthcare in Australia."

approaches that truly support individuals in navigating their health care – as patients, consumers, and persons deserving of comprehensive and dignified care.

Chapter Summary

Moving toward more inclusive health care policy in the United States requires a multifaceted approach that integrates access, equity, and the SDOH. By addressing systemic barriers and fostering culturally competent care, inclusive policies can bridge gaps in health care access and outcomes for marginalized communities. The whole being model emphasizes the need to see individuals not just as patients but also as consumers and persons, balancing clinical needs, financial realities, and lifestyle considerations. This holistic framework enables the creation of policies that align health care delivery with the diverse needs of the population, ultimately promoting trust, engagement, and better health outcomes.

Achieving inclusivity in health care policy will require collaboration across sectors, investment in community health resources, and the integration of technology and mental health services. Policy makers must also prioritize equity-focused legislation, promote workforce diversity, and expand health care coverage to ensure no group is left behind. Drawing lessons from international models, the United States has the opportunity to implement a more integrated system that supports patients comprehensively. By recognizing and addressing the unique challenges faced by underserved populations, inclusive health care policies can foster a system where everyone, regardless of background, has the opportunity to live a healthy, fulfilling life.

CHAPTER 10

Expanding the Role of Patients in Health Care

Insights

- Inclusive health care policies prioritize patient voices, ensuring tailored, culturally competent care that addresses diverse needs and improves outcomes.
- Community-engaged health care (CEH) models are an innovative strategy to drive meaningful community engagement in health care programs and policies.
- Embedding providers in community settings, like pharmacies and retail spaces, reduces barriers and promotes health equity.
- Value-based financial models incentivize preventive care and patient engagement, fostering better health outcomes and cost savings.
- Aligning the interests of the 6 Ps – patients, policy makers, payers, providers, pharmacies, and pharmaceuticals – ensures sustainable, patient-focused health care systems.

Throughout this book, we have utilized the 6 Ps model of health care[1] (Chapter 1) to evaluate the scaling of health care in the United States (Chapter 2), the role of government (Chapter 3), private industry (Chapter 4), health care policy (Chapters 5 and 6), the need for incorporating social determinants (Chapter 7), health equity (Chapter 8), and policies that are inclusive of the people being served in health care, the patients (Chapters 9 and 10). Woven throughout each chapter has been a perspective to prioritize people over politics by emphasizing patient-centered policies, inclusive approaches, and innovative strategies to align health equity with health policy in US health care.

In this chapter, we expand on the roles of patients and providers in their communities and explore financial incentive models that can promote

[1] Gillespie and Privitera, *Patient-Centric Analytics*.

collaboration between these entities. Traditionally, patients have been viewed primarily as passive recipients of care, with their needs and preferences often sidelined during medical decision-making processes. However, the landscape of health care is shifting toward a more participatory model that actively involves patients as essential stakeholders. Patients are increasingly recognized as partners in the decision-making processes that affect their health.[2,3] Empowering patients to openly express their values, perspectives, and preferences can lead to better health outcomes and improved quality of care.[4] This shift therefore parallels the growing emphasis on patient-centric care, which seeks to validate patient experiences and incorporate their voices into treatment plans and health policies to improve patient satisfaction and the overall quality of care.

By expanding patient and provider roles, health care can be more equitable, ensuring that the voices of all patients, particularly those from diverse backgrounds, are heard and considered in the pursuit of optimal health outcomes. Therefore, to emphasize the need for inclusivity and equity in health care, this chapter will begin with a focus on patient-centric care.

10.1 Patient-Centric Care: Community-Engaged Health Care

As discussed throughout this book, patient-centric care has gained significant traction within the health care landscape, emphasizing the critical importance of integrating patients' voices into treatment planning and decision-making. This approach recognizes patients as being active participants in their health care journeys, thereby enhancing engagement and improving clinical outcomes. By valuing and incorporating patients' perspectives, health care providers can deliver more tailored care that meets individual needs, values, and preferences.

Innovative, evidence-based provider practices have been central to advancing patient-centric care and improving health care quality through patient involvement in shared decision-making processes. **Community-engaged health care** is one example of an innovative approach that empowers communities to advocate for their health and design interventions to address their unique needs with support from health providers.[5] The model illustrated in Figure 10.1, published by the National Academy of Medicines' Organizing

---

[2] US Preventive Services Task Force, "Collaboration and Shared Decision-Making."
[3] World Health Organization, "Patient Engagement."
[4] Jiang et al., "Understanding Health Empowerment."
[5] Organizing Committee, "Assessing Meaningful Community Engagement."

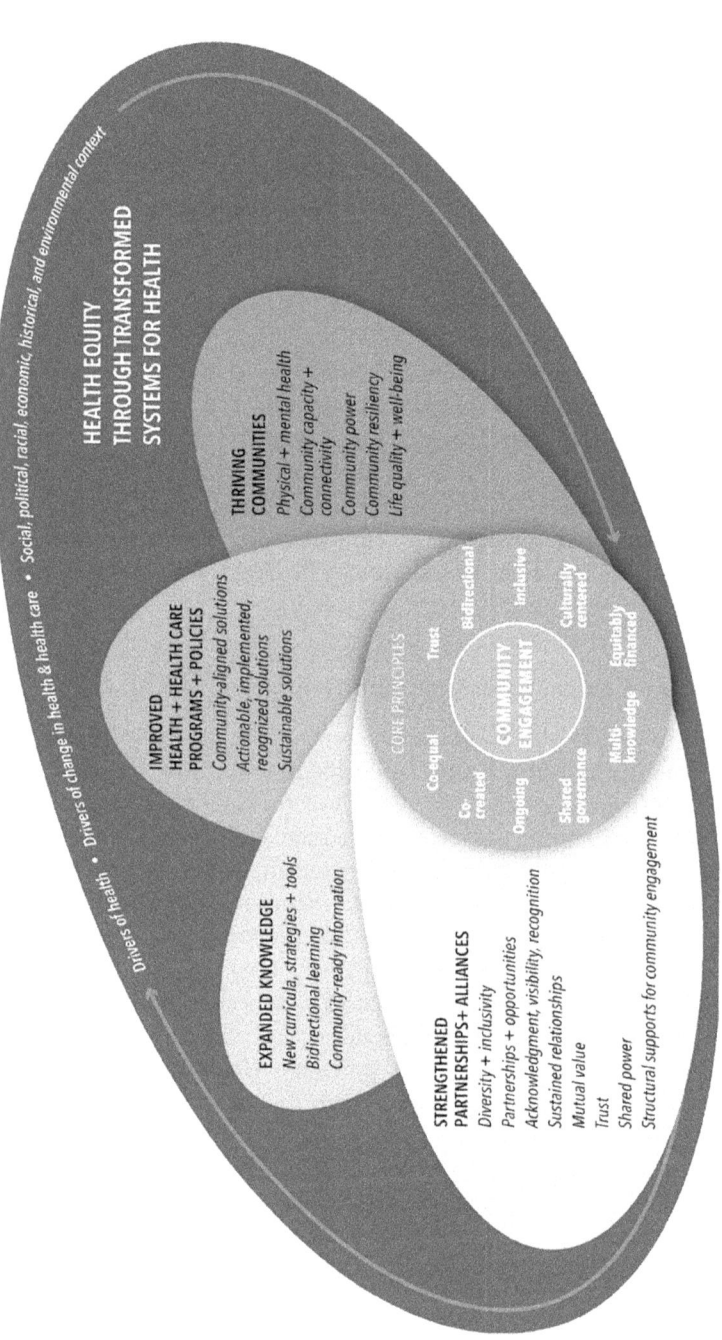

Figure 10.1 Conceptual model to advance health equity through transformed systems for health

Source: Organizing Committee for Assessing Meaningful Community Engagement in Health & Health Care Programs & Policies. 2022. Assessing Meaningful Community Engagement: A Conceptual Model to Advance Health Equity through Transformed Systems for Health. NAM Perspectives. Commentary, National Academy of Medicine, Washington, DC. https://doi.org/10.31478/202202c. Reproduced with permission from the National Academy of Sciences, Courtesy of the National Academies Press, Washington, DC.

Committee for Assessing Meaningful Community Engagement in Health & Health Care Programs & Policies, provides a comprehensive overview of CEH. This model is innovative in that it emphasizes the importance of autonomy and decision-making for patients by shifting power from health care providers to community members, recognizing that traditional health care solutions often fail to address the fundamental issues faced by these populations.[6] This collaborative approach not only addresses health disparities but also fosters trust and strengthens community engagement.

Consider one example of CEH in action, involving the use of community health workers (CHWs) in underserved communities, to improve health outcomes. In this program, CHWs are peers in the community who are trained to provide health education, advocate for and facilitate access to health care resources, and follow up with individuals who miss appointments. Serving as liaisons between health care providers and the community, CHWs have effectively bridged the gap between the health care system and those who often feel alienated from it. This approach allows health care interventions to be tailored to the individual and also to the cultural and social context of the community where they live.

One of the critical components of this initiative is the participatory planning process, which actively involves community members in identifying health priorities and designing interventions that address their specific needs. During community meetings, for example, residents can voice their concerns regarding high rates of chronic diseases and the need for improved mental health support. Using this input, the program can incorporate workshops on diabetes management and mental wellness, thereby responding directly to the expressed needs. The CHWs can go further to organize health fairs, for example, where local health care providers can offer free screenings and consultations in an informal setting to help individuals feel more comfortable receiving their care. These events not only enhance health access but also create a sense of community ownership and responsibility toward health promotion.

10.2 Expanding the Role of Providers: Lessons Learned from the Pandemic

A broader theme from initiatives like the CEH model is to break down misconceptions about how we think about providers or, rather, *who* we think of as providers. Providers are often considered to be doctors or

---

[6] Barker et al., "Community-Engaged Healthcare Model."

physicians who care for those in a hospital or clinic setting. However, as we saw firsthand during the pandemic, this is a restrictive way of viewing providers.[7] During the pandemic in the United States, the role of providers was expanded. States collaborated with the CDC and a wide range of trusted partners to respond to the public health crisis. As vaccine supplies grew, they adapted by setting up large-scale community vaccination clinics, showcasing the flexibility and responsiveness of the public health system to reach all communities. When vaccination rates at traditional health care sites lagged, public health agencies launched large-scale clinics, implemented scheduling systems, extended appointment hours, and created vaccine locator tools. They also partnered with federal retail pharmacy programs to ensure equitable vaccine distribution in long-term care facilities. As the demand for vaccines slowed, partnerships with chain and independent pharmacies expanded to enhance community-based distribution.

The multifaceted approach during the pandemic in the United States did more than demonstrate the value of being adaptive and collaborative in achieving health access and equity; it provided an exemplar for how medicine, and by extension health care, can be delivered in ways that reach people in the very communities where they live, work, and play. For example, it reinforced the expanded role of pharmacies in delivering care, which are much closer to an individual than a hospital, with most people living within 5 miles of a pharmacy, yet over 10 miles away from a hospital, depending on location and rurality.[8] The expanding role of pharmacies, in addressing health equity by *meeting people where they are*, reflects the principle of improving health care delivery by leaning into community-based approaches.

Exploring more broadly, the following strategies to expand the role of providers in health care, which integrate features of the CEH model, can be a strong step toward achieving health equity in health policy:

- *Expanded access through community integration.* Providers are increasingly embedded in diverse settings such as grocery stores, retail chains, and community centers, making health services more convenient and accessible. This expansion ensures that patients can receive care where they live and work, reducing barriers to access.

---

[7] Plescia, Hannan, and Baggett, "COVID-19 Vaccines."
[8] Lam, Broderick, and Toor, "How Far Americans Live."

- *Bridging health disparities.* By offering clinical services like vaccinations, chronic care management, and preventive health measures, providers play a crucial role in reaching populations that may lack access to traditional health care providers. This is especially important for rural, low-income, and underserved areas. When patients receive care by members of their own community, it can foster accountability and trust.
- *Convenience as a driver for equity.* The integration of health services into everyday locations ensures that people who might face challenges such as transportation issues or limited time can still receive essential care. This approach reduces delays in treatment and supports better adherence to care plans.
- *Physicians as trusted health advocates.* Physicians' visibility and accessibility tend to position them as trusted voices in the health care system and in their communities. Their role in education, counseling, and medication management ensures patients are informed and empowered to make decisions about their health.
- *Meeting growing health care demands.* The shortage of traditional health care providers underscores the importance of expanding the scope of physicians' roles. By delivering clinical services, physicians can help address the increasing demand for quality care, particularly in communities with limited resources.
- *Preventive and holistic care delivery.* Pharmacies' growing involvement in areas like vaccination campaigns and medication management supports a more holistic approach to care. This includes improving population health outcomes and reducing the strain on emergency and inpatient care systems.

By embedding care into locations that people frequent and expanding the role of providers, the health care system can better address disparities, promote equity, and deliver high-quality care that is tailored to the needs of diverse populations. This patient-centered approach is a critical step toward creating a more inclusive and effective health care system.

10.3 Aligning the Interests of HCOs and Community Leaders

Collaboration between health care organizations (HCOs) and community leaders is crucial to addressing health disparities and advancing health equity. As health care systems face increasing demands to treat illness and promote wellness, partnerships with local communities can enhance their ability to respond to the unique health needs of diverse populations. Key strategies that can help foster open collaboration between HCOs and community leaders include each of the following:

Building trust through open communication. Trust is the foundation upon which successful collaborations are built. Open communication plays a pivotal role in establishing this trust. Health Care organizations should create spaces for dialogue where community leaders can express their perspectives, challenges, and insights regarding health issues in their communities.[9] Regular meetings, forums, and community-engagement events can facilitate these discussions, allowing for transparency regarding the HCO's goals and operations. For example, community forums can provide opportunities for health care leaders to share information about available services while simultaneously gathering feedback on how those services can meet the real needs of the population. By listening to community input and incorporating it into health care strategies, HCOs can build rapport with community leaders and reinforce their commitment to community health.

Establishing shared goals and mutual respect. A successful partnership hinges on identifying shared goals that reflect the priorities of both HCOs and community leaders. Collaborative initiatives should be designed to address specific health outcomes that have direct relevance to the community, thus ensuring that efforts are meaningful and impactful.[10] For example, if a community faces high rates of diabetes, both parties can work together to develop educational programs focused on prevention and management, nutrition workshops, and access to healthy foods. Moreover, community leaders often possess valuable local knowledge and cultural insights that can inform health care strategies. By recognizing this expertise and involving community leaders in decision-making processes, HCOs can develop culturally competent programs that resonate with community members, fostering mutual respect among stakeholders. This respect creates an environment of partnership, rather than one of service provider versus service recipient.

Leveraging community resources. Health Care organizations can benefit significantly from tapping into existing community resources. Community organizations, local nonprofits, religious institutions, and advocacy groups can provide vital connections to underserved populations. By forming alliances with these entities, health care providers can enhance access to their services and ensure that they reach those who may otherwise remain

---

[9] Lansing et al., "Building Trust."   [10] Ellis et al., "Hospital Organizational Change."

disengaged from the health system.[11] Projects that utilize community resources can lead to collaborative, innovative solutions to health issues. For example, local faith-based organizations can facilitate health education workshops or health fairs, while HCOs can offer expertise, resources, and staff to support these community efforts. This strategy not only increases the reach of health care services but also reinforces community ownership over health initiatives, which is crucial for sustainable change.

Training and capacity building. Investing in training and capacity building for both health care staff and community leaders can enhance collaboration outcomes.[12] By equipping health care staff with an understanding of social determinants of health and community engagement principles, organizations can foster empathy and cultural competence within their teams. This training can result in more informed interactions with community members and improved patient-centered care. Conversely, providing training for community leaders in areas such as health literacy, advocacy, and systems thinking can empower them to be effective partners in health promotion. Programs that focus on developing skills enhance community leaders' ability to influence health decisions and mobilize their communities around important health initiatives. Through collaborative training efforts, both parties can cultivate a shared understanding of challenges and strategies to improve community health outcomes.

Implementing data-driven strategies. Utilizing data to inform partnership strategies can lead to more effective collaborations. Health Care organizations can leverage data analytics to identify health trends, gaps in service delivery, and patient outcomes, which can guide community engagement efforts.[13] Additionally, community leaders can provide qualitative insights that enrich data interpretations, offering a comprehensive understanding of the barriers faced by their constituents. Establishing mechanisms to share data with community partners fosters transparency and encourages joint evaluation of programs. For example, tracking the impact of health initiatives on specific health outcomes can provide both HCOs and community leaders with evidence to refine strategies and advocate for resources. Such data-driven dialogues reinforce accountability and enable informed decision-making regarding health initiatives.

Ultimately, effective collaboration between HCOs and community leaders is essential for advancing health equity and improving health

---

[11] Raday, Chan, and Krodel, "Healthy Outcomes."
[12] Shegaze Shimbre and Tanga, "Collaborative Care."
[13] Thomas Craig et al., "Leveraging Data."

outcomes. The strategies discussed in this section can truly strengthen HCO and community ties by ensuring that they meet the diverse needs of the populations they serve. This integrated approach *meets people where they are* and paves the way for healthier communities, thereby enhancing the quality of life for all individuals within those communities.

10.4 Exploring Innovation for Financial Incentive Models

The dynamic landscape of health care increasingly prompts the need for addressing a pivotal component in achieving inclusive care: the financial incentive systems shaping health care delivery. This section explores the current state of financial incentives in health care, examines proposed reforms to align these models with patient-centered values, and analyzes successful examples that reward preventive care and health outcomes – while also addressing the associated challenges and opportunities.

Traditional financial incentive models in health care focus primarily on system efficiency, often evaluating performance based on the volume of services rendered rather than the quality or effectiveness of care delivered. This fee-for-service (FFS) structure can inadvertently prioritize quantity over quality, leading to an increase in unnecessary procedures and a neglect of holistic patient well-being. Such models have resulted in fragmented care experiences, where patients often feel like mere statistics in a system that is focused more on financial outputs than on their specific health needs.[14] Health Care systems operating under these models often prioritize short-term cost savings, leading to a reactive rather than proactive approach to patient management. This focus detracts from preventive care initiatives and long-term health outcomes, as the financial incentives do not align with efforts to enhance patient engagement or improve overall health. Instead, the emphasis tends to lie on short-lived financial gain rather than on fostering sustainable health improvements among patients.

Recognizing the limitations of traditional incentive models, practical steps should be taken for reshaping financial incentives to better align with patient-centered values. These include integrating quality metrics into reimbursement models, wherein providers are rewarded not just for services rendered but also for their effectiveness in improving patient outcomes. By establishing incentive structures that reward the delivery of high-quality, patient-centered care, HCOs can encourage providers to invest in preventive measures and improve patient outcomes and engagement.

---

[14] Wang et al., "Fee-for-Service."

10.4 Innovation for Financial Incentive Models

A significant rethinking of how value is defined within the health care ecosystem could be beneficial, to advocate for a more comprehensive approach that encompasses patient satisfaction, adherence to care plans, and health outcomes.[15] Assessment of patient experiences would then be critical to determining financial incentives. Implementing **patient-reported outcome measures** as a cornerstone of performance evaluation, for example, can support this transition, ensuring that patient perspectives are fundamental in assessing health care quality and financial reimbursement. Such an approach not only enhances accountability but also fosters a culture that is centered on patient experiences, ultimately driving higher satisfaction rates and improved health outcomes.

The health care sector has witnessed the emergence of innovative financial incentive models that have successfully integrated patient-centered ideals with effective health care delivery. One such model is the **Accountable Care Organization (ACO)**, where health care providers are given shared financial responsibility for the care of a defined patient population. Collaboration among providers is incentivized by ACOs, focusing on population health management that promotes preventive care and long-term health outcomes while providing avenues for cost savings. Moreover, various value-based care programs reward providers based on their ability to meet specific quality metrics and health outcomes, often linked to adherence to care plans and preventive services. For example, initiatives that provide bonuses to physicians for meeting patient-engagement benchmarks, such as regular followups or encouraging preventive screenings, demonstrate the potential of rewarding positive behaviors. These models not only improve patient health but also reduce overall health care costs, reaffirming the viability of a patient-centric financial incentive approach.[16]

In the contemporary health care environment, incentivizing patients through financial means has emerged as a pivotal strategy to promote healthier behaviors and enhance engagement in preventive care.[17] The premise of paying patients to encourage healthy behavior is grounded in economic theories that suggest financial rewards can modify individual behavior.[18] By offering monetary or other incentives for participating in preventive care measures, such as regular checkups, screenings, and adherence to treatment plans, HCOs can reduce barriers that may

---

[15] Gillespie and Privitera, "Bringing Patient Incentives."
[16] Krist et al., "Engaging Patients."
[17] Gillespie and Privitera, "Bringing Patient Incentives."
[18] Vlaev et al., "Changing Health Behaviors."

Collaborative goal-setting between patient and provider	Build incentive programs with resource allocation	Immediate reward for goal achievement; reset goals or adjust goals based on outcome
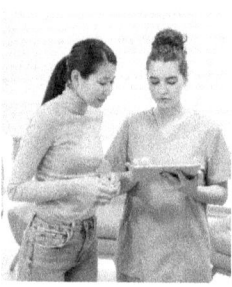	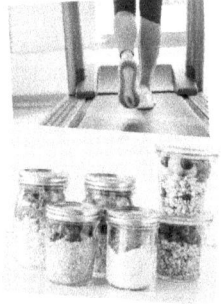	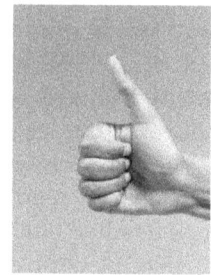
Set health goal: for example, weight loss. Metric can be pre-post weight or body mass index (BMI) score to assess progress	Provide resources to support goal attainment. For example, provide informational pamphlets, time with a nutritionist, or access to exercise	Offer immediate reward upon goal attainment. Examples of incentives: gift cards, hotel stays, $0 copay, or even cash

Figure 10.2 Personalizing rewards using good target incentives for patients to reach health goals
Source: Left photo, A doctor and a patient looking at a tablet by Cedric Fauntleroy. Top-center photo, Person using a treadmill by Andrea Piacquadio. Bottom-center photo, Six fruit cereals in clear glass jars by Ella Olsson. Right photo, person doing a thumbs up by Rocketmann Team.

otherwise prevent individuals from seeking care. The structure of such a model, using **good target incentives**, is illustrated in Figure 10.2.

Good target incentives include: avoiding early-onset diabetes, quitting tobacco, controlling cholesterol, lowering blood pressure, and reducing weight. Setting good target incentives between patient and provider can be used to build incentive regimes for patients to learn more, take action, and become/stay healthier. Examples of incentive programs include those offering small cash incentives for completing preventive screenings or attending wellness visits, gift cards as rewards for engaging in preventive health behaviors, lowering copay costs for preventive services to make them more accessible, and combining incentives with educational initiatives to promote understanding of preventive care.[19] This approach presents opportunities for meaningful community outreach by fostering partnerships between local community leaders and businesses with HCOs (e.g., having local businesses promote participation by offering good target

---
[19] County Health Rankings & Roadmaps, "Patient Financial Incentives."

incentives) and connecting with patients on a personal or cultural level by tailoring incentive programs for each individual patient.

Using financial incentive models for patients requires understanding the psychosocial factors that influence patients' health decisions, such that immediate financial rewards can bridge the gap between inconvenience and the long-term benefits of preventive care. This approach not only promotes personal health management, but can also alleviate some of the financial burdens associated with preventive services. Important considerations include tailoring incentives that are culturally sensitive and relevant, ensuring that incentives are accessible and understandable to the individual, and evaluating and monitoring the effectiveness of incentive programs to evolve these programs over time.

While the transition to patient-centric financial incentives opens up significant opportunities, it also poses challenges that HCOs must navigate. One primary challenge lies in balancing cost efficiency with patient engagement and satisfaction. As health care providers strive to implement comprehensive care programs, they may face resistance to change, particularly from stakeholders accustomed to traditional FFS models. Additionally, the integration of new metrics and quality measures can create initial complexities in data management, requiring robust analytics and reporting systems to evaluate progress effectively and accurately.

Nevertheless, the potential to improve both patient outcomes and satisfaction levels provides a compelling incentive for HCOs to invest in adapting their financial models. There are significant opportunities for harnessing technology, such as telehealth and patient-engagement apps, to facilitate knowledge-sharing and establish ongoing communication between HCOs and patients. By focusing on building trust and enhancing patient relationships, HCOs can bridge the gap between cost efficiency and patient satisfaction, achieving a balance that promotes holistic, inclusive health care approaches.

10.5 Across the Pond: Putting People over Politics

Across the health care ecosystem, aligning the interests of various stakeholders is vital for fostering an effective and patient-centered system. While leveraging international comparisons to inform discussions on care throughout this text, the landscape of health care in the United States is discussed largely through the lens of the 6 Ps model, which encompasses patients, policy makers, pharmacies, pharmaceuticals, payers, and providers. By aligning interests across the 6 Ps, we can enhance patient engagement, improve health outcomes, and create a more sustainable health care policy that rightfully puts patients at the center of the health care model. In this closing section, we advocate for actionable change among key stakeholders, and for health policy that empowers patients in our health care systems.

The benefits of expanding patient roles resonate at the individual, provider, and community levels. Engaged patients are healthier and experience better outcomes as they take greater control over their health decisions, participate actively in treatment plans, and manage chronic conditions more effectively. This personal investment not only leads to tangible health benefits for patients, such as reduced hospital admissions and lower health care costs, but also enhances their overall satisfaction with the health care experience. Furthermore, when patients are actively involved, providers benefit from improved adherence to treatment recommendations and increased loyalty/trust, which are crucial for long-term practice sustainability.[20]

At the community level, fostering patient engagement bolsters public health initiatives through increased participation in preventive care and chronic disease management. Building a health care system that promotes inclusivity creates a positive feedback loop, where communities become empowered to address health challenges collaboratively, thus reducing health disparities and strengthening trust for delivering health care in those communities. By recognizing and harnessing the potential of active patient participation and overall collaboration across the 6 Ps, we can transform health care delivery into a more collaborative and efficient process that benefits everyone involved.[21]

To realize the vision of a patient-inclusive health care system, a concerted effort among stakeholders – the 6 Ps – is essential. By aligning interests across the 6 Ps model and actively engaging patients at the individual, provider, and community levels, we can foster more effective and sustainable health care at a systems and policy level. The collective responsibility falls on prioritizing this alignment through meaningful collaboration. Future research and technological advancements will further empower patients, paving the way for a health care landscape that truly puts patients at the center of the system that was designed to serve them. The message is clear: Let us work together to design an inclusive environment that benefits everyone involved in the health care journey. The best way to reach all Americans is through bipartisan policy that puts *people before politics*.

---

[20] Marzban et al., "Impact of Patient Engagement."
[21] Durrance-Bagale et al., "Community Engagement."

Chapter Summary

This book has presented a comprehensive framework for reimagining health care systems, rooted in the principle that optimizing the health of all people must extend beyond the health care system itself. From the foundational 6 Ps model introduced in Chapter 1, to exploring global comparisons, government and private-sector roles, the integration of social determinants, and the pursuit of health equity, each chapter has aligned data with exemplar international comparisons to identify the value of patient-centered, inclusive care. Central to this vision is the idea that health care policy should put *people before politics*, advocating for solutions that align access, quality, and cost with the needs of the populations being served.

In the final chapters, the whole being model and innovative patient incentive strategies reinforced the importance of empowering patients to be active participants in their care. By embracing empathy, cultural competence, and meaningful engagement, health care systems can humanize the experience for patients, ensuring they are treated as more than recipients of care, but as essential stakeholders. As we close, the message is to treat health care as it was intended: to serve *all* people. Achieving an optimal health care system requires bipartisan solutions, collaboration across sectors, and a commitment to addressing health disparities at their roots. Through the alignment of interests across the 6 Ps and a steadfast focus on equity, we can foster a health care system that serves all people, ensuring that health is a right, not a privilege, and that every individual has the opportunity to thrive.

Glossary

6 Ps pentagonal framework for health care A framework for understanding the health care ecosystem in which each sector or entity in the health care system is represented by the 6 Ps: patients, policy makers, providers, pharmacies, pharmaceuticals, and payers. (1)

Beveridge model A health care system in which the government acts as the single-payer, providing health care coverage for all citizens through income tax payments. (1)

Bismarck model A health care system characterized by mandatory employer and employee contributions through payroll deductions to fund health insurance plans. (1)

Bloomberg Global Health Index A comprehensive measure of national health that includes many factors such as health risks (e.g., obesity) average life expectancy, and living conditions (e.g., water quality); it is scored as a value between 0 and 100, with larger values indicating better health. (1)

Donabedian model Healthcare quality measures developed by Avedis Donabedian that are classified into three categories: structure, process, and outcome; the structure of health care influences the processes of care, which, in turn, influence the effect of care on health status. (1)

Equality The even distribution of resources to address inequality in a system. (1)

Equity The custom distribution of resources to uniquely address inequality in a system for each individual. (1)

Fractionalization Index A measure of the likelihood that two people, selected at random, in a given population, will be from two different groups; it is scored as a value between 0 and 100, with larger values indicating greater diversity for a given measure. (1)

Healthcare Access and Quality Index (HAQ) A comprehensive measure based on death rates from thirty-two causes of death that could be avoided with proper medical care that is used to evaluate and compare the quality of national health care access; the HAQ is measured on a scale from 0 (least accessible) to 100 (most accessible). (1)

Justice The equitable treatment of persons in a system that includes fixing inequalities in that system. (1)

Glossary

National Health Insurance Model A health care system that combines the aspects of the Beveridge and Bismarck models, with the government acting as a single-payer, while providers remain private. (1)

Out-of-pocket model The model of health care characterized by the absence of a formalized health care system, in which individuals must pay for their own medical expenses out-of-pocket. (1)

Copay A fixed amount, specified by a health insurance plan, that covered patients are required to pay for certain medical services or prescriptions at the time of care; they facilitate cost sharing between insurer and insured. (2)

Deductible The amount of money a patient must pay directly, out of pocket, for health care services before their medical insurance begins to cover costs; these can vary widely in amounts, with some levels of deductibles potentially imposing financial hardship on patients. (2)

Employer-provided insurance Plans to cover a range of medical services that employers provide to employees as part of a benefits package; they vary substantially in cost, coverage, and provider networks, often including contributions from the employee to help offset costs and build in proper incentives for utilization. (2)

Frequent flyers The patients who, due to poor management of health care issues, limited access to primary care, or chronic conditions and comorbidities, are heavy users of health care services, often visiting emergency rooms and hospitals several times within a brief period. (2)

Primary care physician (PCP) A medical doctor serving as the first point of contact for patients and providing comprehensive health care, typically with a focus on overall health, disease prevention, initial diagnosis, and coordinating specialist referrals. (2)

Coinsurance The proportion of costs for covered health care services that a health plan requires patients to pay before the deductible is met; the insurer may pay 80 percent of the costs while the patient is responsible for 20 percent, or for example, the percentage allocation could be 90–10 percent. (3)

Community health worker (CHW) A trained professional who serves as a bridge between communities/patients and health care providers, helping provide education, information, improved access, and overall system navigation; they can help promote health equity and reduce disparities faced by underserved populations. (3)

Health Professional Shortage Area (HPSA) A region or population that has an insufficient number of health care providers to effectively meet the needs of a community, resulting in longer wait times, limited access to specialists, skipped care, and higher rates of disparities/inequalities. (3)

Health-related social needs (HRSN) The social factors (e.g., food security, housing stability, physical safety, social support, and transportation access) that impact an individual's health and wellness; they emphasize the interconnectedness of positive health outcomes and social determinants. (3)

Insurance premium The amount paid regularly (e.g., monthly, quarterly, or annually) by an individual or company/organization to an insurer in exchange for health care coverage; these payments vary depending on the insurer's underwriting guidelines, the insured person's risk profile, and the level of coverage attained. (3)

Medically Underserved Area/Population (MUA/MUP) A region or population that lacks consistent access to comprehensive health care services due to economic disadvantage, geographic isolation, or paucity of providers. (3)

Negative externality A situation where the actions of one entity have adverse effects and costs that are at least partially transferred onto other entities, leading to economic distortions and market failures that typically require some form of intervention to mitigate their negative impact. (3)

Over-the-counter (OTC) medicine The medication that can be purchased without a prescription from a physician or other health care provider; when used according to the labeling, they are considered convenient, effective, and safe for treating common problems such as allergies, colds, headaches, nausea, and sleeplessness. (3)

Positive externality A situation where the actions of one entity have favorable effects and benefits that are at least partially transferred onto other entities, leading to economic distortions and market failures that typically require some form of intervention to maximize their positive impact. (3)

School-based health center (SBHC) A health care facility that improves access to medical services for children and adolescents by colocating in or near K-12 schools; they are often essential for allowing students to access convenient care without missing too many classes. (3)

Universal health care coverage (UHC) A nationwide system providing all individuals with access to essential health services including education, preventive care, diagnosis, treatment, and rehabilitation, regardless of their income or socioeconomic status, so patients pay little or zero directly, avoiding financial hardships and the need go without coverage/care. (3)

Essential Packages of Health Services (EPHS) The prioritized health services (e.g., child and maternal health, infectious diseases, and preventive care) considered necessary to meet the most pressing health needs of a population, especially in resource-limited populations or settings. (4)

Medicaid A joint federal and state health insurance program, adopted in 1965 in the United States, and designed for eligible low-income individuals and families. It covers a wide range of health services, emergency rooms, hospital stays, long-term care, physician visits, and preventive care. The eligibility criteria (e.g., family size, income level, disability, pregnancy) vary substantially by state. (4)

Medicare A federal health insurance program, adopted in 1965 in the United States, and designed for individuals aged sixty-five and older, as well as those with disabilities or specific diseases. It consists of several parts: Part A covers hospital insurance, Part B covers medical insurance, Part C (Medicare Advantage) offers a way to gain Medicare benefits via private insurance plans, and Part D covers prescription drugs. (4)

Medicare Advantage Also known as Part C, a health insurance plan offered by private companies contracting with Medicare to provide benefits, typically including the original Medicare benefits (Part A, Part B, and Part D) and additional services such as dental and vision. These plans often have different costs, coverage rules, and provider networks than regular Medicare. (4)

Private health provider (PHP) An individual or organization (e.g., private hospitals, clinics, specialists, and physician practices) operating independently of government funding or public health systems; they offer a full range of medical services and typically receive payment from patients directly or through private health insurance plans. (4)

Public–private partnership (PPP) A collaborative agreement between government entities, nongovernmental organizations, and private-sector companies to more successfully complete large projects by incorporating new perspectives, leveraging differing experience/expertise, and sharing costs/risks. (4)

Urgent care clinic A health care facility providing immediate, nonemergency medical attention for a variety of conditions (typically, relatively minor illnesses and injuries such as flu-like symptoms, headaches, infections, soreness, and sprains) and serving as an alternative to the high cost and longer wait times of emergency departments. (4)

Data interoperability The ability of different health care information systems and software applications to communicate, exchange, aggregate, and leverage information effectively across various organizations, platforms, and systems. By expanding the availability of data for descriptive, predictive, and prescriptive analytics, it helps enhance overall patient outcomes, improve care coordination, increase diagnosis accuracy, and reduce medical errors. (5)

Fee-for-service A traditional health care delivery/payment model where providers are reimbursed for each specific medical service performed (e.g., treatments, tests, visits), incentivizing generation of higher volumes to maximize revenue, with potentially less focus on patient outcomes and care quality. It is often contrasted with value-based care models. (5)

Internet of Medical Things (IoMT) The interconnected network of medical applications, software, and devices (e.g., mobile health applications, smart medical equipment, and wearable health monitors) that communicate and exchange data over the internet. It can improve organizational management and patient care by facilitating more effective utilization of data for real-time and long-term decision-making. (5)

Remote patient monitoring (RPM) Uses technology to monitor health data remotely, typically originating from the patient's home, allowing real-time data collection on symptoms, vital signs, and overall health status without the inconvenience of in-person visits. By enabling timely interventions, it can enhance patient engagement, improve chronic condition management, and reduce hospital admissions. (5)

Value-based care A relatively new health care delivery/payment model incentivizing providers to maximize patient health outcomes and the quality of care instead of service volume; innovative structures include bundled payments, capitation contracts, and shared savings programs. It is often contrasted with fee-for-service models. (5)

Veterans Affairs Health System (VA) A comprehensive health care system, operated by the US Department of Veterans Affairs, providing a wide range of medical services to eligible military veterans, particularly for unique mental and physical health challenges related to military service. (5)

Centers for Medicare & Medicaid Services (CMS) A US agency within the federal Department of Health and Human Services (HHS) that administers key health care programs, including Medicare, Medicaid, and the Children's Health Insurance Program (CHIP), with the goals being to improve access, increase quality, reduce costs, and promote innovation. (6)

Healthcare abuse The adverse practices resulting in unnecessary costs to the health care system, the ones that stop short of being outrightly fraudulent and illegal. Examples include overutilization of services, ordering duplicative or unnecessary tests or treatments, providing substandard care, and upcoding to achieve higher reimbursement. Along with fraud and waste, it can lead to increased health care costs, negative patient outcomes, and reduced system integrity. (6)

Healthcare fraud The adverse practices designed to obtain unauthorized benefits or payments from health care insurers or programs, typically describing conduct that is both deceptive and illegal. Examples include billing for products or services never provided, double billing, inflating costs/prices, and providing completely unnecessary medical treatments. Along with abuse and waste, it can lead to increased health care costs, negative patient outcomes, and reduced system integrity. (6)

Healthcare waste The adverse practices resulting in unnecessary or inefficient use of resources in a health care organization or system, resulting in excessive costs. Examples include duplication of administrative work, inappropriate disposal of hazardous items, overuse of medical services, and waste of medical supplies. Along with abuse and fraud, it can lead to increased health care costs, negative patient outcomes, and reduced system integrity. (6)

Medical loss ratio (MLR) The percentage of insurance premium dollars that health insurance companies spend on direct health services and medical care for their members versus expenditures on administrative costs and their residual profits. (6)

Health equity The custom distribution of resources, in a health care system, to uniquely address inequality for each individual. (7)

Medication adherence The extent to which a person's actions correspond with or follow the agreed-upon recommendations from a health care provider. (7)

Organisation for Economic Co-operation and Development (OECD) A forum consisting of thirty-seven governmental democracies with market-based economies that collaborate to develop policy standards to promote sustainable economic growth. (7)

Glossary

Social determinants of health (SDOH) The lived environments where people are born, live, learn, work, play, worship, and age that can affect the health of an individual or population. (7)

Wrong pockets problem A problem that arises in reimbursement when one entity makes investments to improve a social condition while another entity accrues those same benefits. (7)

Food insecurity A condition experienced by a person or household with limited, uncertain, or unstable access to nutritionally adequate and safe foods. (8)

Systemic barriers Obstacles, regulations, and structures, often ingrained in organizations, that deny people or groups access to resources and opportunities necessary for their complete engagement in society. (8)

Accountable Health Communities (AHC) model Launched by the Centers for Medicare & Medicaid Services (CMS), it is a model to improve health outcomes for Medicare and Medicaid beneficiaries by identifying and addressing nonmedical factors that influence health. (9)

Children's Health Insurance Program (CHIP) A program designed to provide health insurance to uninsured children from families that earn too much money to qualify for Medicaid, but cannot afford private coverage. (9)

Cultural Competency Training initiative Trainings developed by the US Department of Health and Human Services (HHS) to meet the needs of culturally diverse populations by offering a range of training programs on cultural competence in health care. (9)

Federally Qualified Health Centers (FQHCs) Community-based, nonprofit health care centers that receive federal funding to deliver primary care services, including telehealth services and community outreach to underserved populations in the United States. (9)

Health Center Program A national network of community health centers in the United States that provide comprehensive and affordable care, irrespective of patients' ability to pay. (9)

Health Literacy Action Plan A strategic approach in the United States, developed by the CDC, to promote health literacy as part of inclusive health policy; the plan outlines specific goals and strategies aimed at improving health literacy across diverse groups. (9)

Human Rights Campaign's Healthcare Equality Index (HEI) Provides a framework for health care facilities to assess their policies and practices concerning LGBTQ+ patient care. (9)

Inclusive health care A system of health care that thoroughly integrates principles of equity and accessibility in all levels of health care delivery. (9)

Mental Health Parity and Addiction Equity Act (MHPAEA) Legislation in the United States that ensures that individuals who have group health plans or individual health insurance who seek treatment for covered mental health or substance-use disorders do not face greater burdens to access benefits for those conditions or disorders than they would face when seeking coverage for the treatment of a medical condition or a surgical procedure. (9)

National Health Service Corps (NHSC) Policy designed in the United States to improve access to primary health care in areas experiencing shortages of health care providers, particularly in rural and low-income urban areas, by incentivizing health professionals to practice in underserved communities through scholarships, recruitment, community engagement, and training. (9)

Older Americans Act (OAA) A model for expanding resources and care options that prioritize inclusivity and cultural sensitivity in geriatric care. (9)

Patient-Centered Medical Home (PCMH) An approach in the United States to delivering high-quality, cost-effective primary care that is patient-centered, culturally appropriate, and team-based to coordinate patient care across a health system. (9)

Patients' Bill of Rights A list of rights and responsibilities for patients, recognized by the US Department of State's Bureau of Medical Services. (9)

Telehealth The use of telecommunication technologies to deliver health care remotely. (9)

Whole being model A framework for humanizing individuals as being more than just *patients* within the health care ecosystem by describing individuals across three dimensions or roles: the patient, the consumer, and the person. (9)

Accountable Care Organization (ACO) A group of health care providers that share financial responsibility for the care of a defined patient population. (10)

Community-Engaged Healthcare (CEH) An approach that empowers communities to advocate for their health and design interventions to address their unique needs with support from health providers. (10)

Good target incentives Personalized incentives allocated to patients for reaching shared health goals agreed upon by the provider and patient. (10)

Patient-reported outcome measures (PROMs) Measures that utilize standardized survey tools to determine the short- or long-term impact of a therapy, patient interaction, or an intervention, by comparing pre- and post-event surveys. (10)

Bibliography

111th Congress. *H.R. 3590 – Patient Protection and Affordable Care Act.* March 23, 2010. www.govinfo.gov.

116th Congress. *H.R.8436 – Equal Health Care for All Act.* October 1, 2020. www.congress.gov/bill/116th-congress/house-bill/8436/text.

ABC123. "The Failed Launch of www.HealthCare.gov." *Harvard Business School Digital Initiative,* November 18, 2016. https://d3.harvard.edu.

Abersone, Ilze. "Patient Advocacy: The Growing Voice of Healthcare." *International Society for Pharmacoeconomics and Outcomes Research (ISPOR)* 8, no. 1 (2022): 20–23. http://bit.ly/3Tri8nD.

Administration for Community Living. *Older Americans Act.* Last modified October 31, 2023. https://acl.gov.

Agency for Healthcare Research and Quality. *2023 National Healthcare Quality and Disparities Report Appendixes.* December 2023. www.ahrq.gov.

Agency for Healthcare Research and Quality. *Executive Summary.* Last modified September 2020. www.ahrq.gov.

Ahmad, Farida B., Jodi A. Cisewski, and Robert N. Anderson. "Mortality in the United States – Provisional Data, 2023." *Morbidity and Mortality Weekly Report* 73, no. 31 (2024): 677–681. http://doi.org/10.15585/mmwr.mm7331a1.

American Health Information Management Association Foundation. "Health Equity and Broadband Internet Access." Last modified February 9, 2023. https://ahimafoundation.ahima.org.

American Hospital Association. "AHA Report: Rural Hospital Closures Threaten Patient Access to Care." Last modified September 8, 2022. www.aha.org.

American Medical Association. "Trends in Health Care Spending." Last modified July 9, 2024. www.ama-assn.org.

Anawade, Pankajkumar A., Deepak Sharma, and Shailesh Gahane. "A Comprehensive Review on Exploring the Impact of Telemedicine on Healthcare Accessibility." *Cureus* 16, no. 3 (2024): e55996. http://doi.org/10.7759/cureus.55996.

Archer, Diane. "Medicare Is More Efficient than Private Insurance." *Health Affairs* (blog), September 20, 2011. www.healthaffairs.org.

Arnaout, Angel, Melina Oseguera-Arasmou, Nikesh Mishra et al. "Leveraging Technology in Public-Private Partnerships: A Model to Address Public Health

Inequities." *Frontiers in Health Services* 3 (2023): e1187306. http://doi.org/10.3389/frhs.2023.1187306.

Association of American Medical Colleges. "AAMC Report Reinforces Mounting Physician Shortage." Last modified June 11, 2021. www.aamc.org.

Authenticx. "Actively Listening to Voice of the Customer at Scale." Accessed December 26, 2024. https://authenticx.com.

Ayanian, John Z., Joel S. Weissman, Eric C. Schneider, Jack A. Ginsburg, and Alan M. Zaslavsky. "Unmet Health Needs of Uninsured Adults in the United States." *JAMA* 284, no. 16 (2000): 2061–2069. http://doi.org/10.1001/jama.284.16.2061.

Baich, Kim. "Understanding Health Inequalities." *Pan Foundation*, May 5, 2023. www.panfoundation.org.

Bailey, Peggy. "Housing and Health Partners Can Work Together to Close the Housing Affordability Gap." *Center on Budget and Policy Priorities*, January 17, 2020. www.cbpp.org.

Baradaran, Dominique. "Community Health Workers Meet People Where They Are to Build Trust, Elevate Voices, and Address Health Disparities in Higher-Risk Communities." *NACCHO*, August 10, 2023. www.naccho.org.

Barker, Stephanie L., Nick Maguire, Robin E. Gearing et al. "Community-Engaged Healthcare Model for Currently Under-Served Individuals Involved in the Healthcare System." *Science Direct* 15 (2021): 100905. http://doi.org/10.1016/j.ssmph.2021.100905.

Barnett, Michael L., Ellen Meara, Terri Lewinson et al. "Racial Inequality in Receipt of Medications for Opioid Use Disorder." *New England Journal of Medicine* 388, no. 19 (2023): 1779–1789. http://doi.org/10.1056/NEJMsa2212412.

Berg, Sara. "What Doctors Wish Patients Knew about Falling U.S. Life Expectancy." *American Medical Association*, March 10, 2023. www.ama-assn.org.

Berger, Simone, Ana Maria Saut, and Fernando Tobal Berssaneti. "Using Patient Feedback to Drive Quality Improvement in Hospitals: A Qualitative Study." *BMJ Open* 10, no. 10 (2020): e037641. https://doi.org/10.1136/bmjopen-2020-037641.

Berlin, Gretchen, Meredith Lapointe, Mhoire Murphy, and Joanna Wexler. "Assessing the Lingering Impact of COVID-19 on the Nursing Workforce." *McKinsey & Company*, May 11, 2022. www.mckinsey.com.

Best, Matthew J., Edward G. McFarland, Savyasachi C. Thakkar, and Uma Srikumaran. "Racial Disparities in the Use of Surgical Procedures in the US." *JAMA Surgery* 156, no. 3 (2021): 274–281. http://doi.org/10.1001/jamasurg.2020.6257.

Beyene, Sisay Demissew. "The Impact of Food Insecurity on Health Outcomes: Empirical Evidence from Sub-Saharan African Countries." *BMC Public Health* 23, no. 388 (2023): 338. https://doi.org/10.1186/s12889-023-15244-3.

Bipartisan Policy Center. "The Future of Health Care." Accessed December 20, 2024. https://bipartisanpolicy.org.

Blair, Jenny. "Study: More than 335,000 Lives Could Have Been Saved during Pandemic if U.S. Had Universal Health Care." *Yale School of Public Health*, June 20, 2022. https://ysph.yale.edu.

Blumenthal, David, Evan D. Gumas, Arnav Shah, Munira Z. Gunja, and Reginald D. Williams II. "Mirror, Mirror 2024: A Portrait of the Failing U.S. Health System." *Commonwealth Fund*, September 19, 2024. https://doi.org/10.26099/taog-zp66.

Board of Governors of the Federal Reserve System. *Economic Well-Being of U.S. Households in 2023*. May 2024. https://doi.org/10.17016/8960.

Bonica, Adam, Howard Rosenthal, Kristy Blackwood, and David J. Rothman. "Ideological Sorting of Physicians in Both Geography and the Workplace." *Journal of Health Politics, Policy and Law* 45, no. 6 (2020): 1023–1057. https://doi.org/10.1215/03616878-8641555.

Briesacher, Becky, Rhona Limcangco, and Darrell Gaskin. "Racial and Ethnic Disparities in Prescription Coverage and Medication Use." *Health Care Financing Review* 25, no. 2 (2003): 63–76. https://pubmed.ncbi.nlm.nih.gov/15124378/.

Bulman-Pozen, Jessica. "Partisan Federalism." *Columbia Law School*, 2014. https://scholarship.law.columbia.edu.

Busch, Isolde M., Francesca Moretti, Giulia Travaini, Albert W. Wu, and Michela Rimondini. "Humanization of Care: Key Elements Identified by Patients, Caregivers, and Healthcare Providers. A Systematic Review." *Patient* 12 (2019): 461–474. https://doi.org/10.1007/s40271-019-00370-1.

Busse, Reinhard, Miriam Blümel, Franz Knieps, and Till Bärnighausen. "Statutory Health Insurance in Germany: A Health System Shaped by 135 Years of Solidarity, Self-Governance, and Competition." *Lancet* 390, no. 10097 (2017): 882–897. https://doi.org/10.1016/s0140-6736(17)31280-1.

Butler, Stuart M. "How 'Wrong Pockets' Hurt Health." *JAMA Forum*, August 22, 2018. https://jamanetwork.com.

Butler, Stuart M. "Optimizing Investment in Housing as a Social Determinant of Health." *JAMA Health Forum* 3, no. 9 (2022): e223626. http://doi.org/10.1001/jamahealthforum.2022.3626.

Butler, Stuart M. "Social Spending, Not Medical Spending, Is Key to Health." *Brookings Institution*, July 13, 2016. www.brookings.edu.

Butler, Stuart M. "The Future of the Affordable Care Act: Reassessment and Revision." *JAMA* 316, no. 5 (2016): 495–497. http://doi.org/10.1001/jama.2016.9881.

Carnegie, Dale. *How to Win Friends and Influence People*. Simon and Schuster, 1936.

Center for Health Law and Policy Innovation. "Food Is Medicine." Accessed December 12, 2024. https://chlpi.org.

Center for Healthcare Quality and Payment Reform. "The Crisis in Rural Health Care." Accessed December 6, 2024. https://ruralhospitals.chqpr.org/.

Centers for Disease Control and Prevention (CDC). "Ambulatory Care Use and Physician Office Visits." Last modified April 15, 2024. www.cdc.gov.

Centers for Disease Control and Prevention (CDC). *Communicating about Health Equity Concepts (CHEC)*. Last modified March 23, 2024. www.cdc.gov.

Centers for Disease Control and Prevention (CDC). *National Ambulatory Medical Care Survey: 2018 National Summary Tables*. Accessed December 20, 2024. www.cdc.gov.

Centers for Medicare & Medicaid Services. *Access to Health Coverage*. Last modified December 3, 2024. www.cms.gov.

Centers for Medicare & Medicaid Services. *Health Equity*. Last modified November 5, 2024. www.cms.gov.

Centers for Medicare & Medicaid Services. *Health Related Social Needs*. Accessed December 7, 2024. www.medicaid.gov.

Centers for Medicare & Medicaid Services. "NHE Fact Sheet." Last modified June 12, 2024. www.cms.gov.

Chung, Mimi. "Health Care Reform: Learning from Other Major Health Care Systems." *Princeton Public Health Review*, December 2017. https://pphr.princeton.edu.

Clair, Kiran, Jenny Chang, Argyrios Ziogas et al. "Disparities by Race, Socioeconomic Status, and Insurance Type in the Receipt of NCCN Guideline Concordant Care for Select Cancer Types in California." *Journal of Clinical Oncology* 38, no. 15 (2020): 7031. https://doi.org/10.1200/JCO.2020.38.15_suppl.7031.

Clarke, David. "Harnessing Private Sector Collaboration for Universal Health Coverage." *International Finance Corporation*, October 2, 2024. www.ifc.org.

Cohen, Joshua T., Peter J. Neumann, and Milton C. Weinstein. "Does Preventive Care Save Money? Health Economics and the Presidential Candidates." *New England Journal of Medicine* 358, no. 7 (2008): 661–663. https://doi.org/10.1056/nejmp0708558.

Congressional Budget Office. *Federal Subsidies for Health Insurance: 2023 to 2033*. September 28, 2023. www.cbo.gov.

Congressional Budget Office. *Health Insurance and Its Federal Subsidies: CBO and JCT's May 2023 Baseline Projections*. September 2023. www.cbo.gov.

Coronado, Fátima, Angela J. Beck, Gulzar Shah et al. "Understanding the Dynamics of Diversity in the Public Health Workforce." *Journal of Public Health Management & Practice* 26, no. 4 (2020): 389–392. http://doi.org/10.1097/PHH.0000000000001075.

County Health Rankings & Roadmaps. "Patient Financial Incentives for Preventive Care." Last modified February 7, 2018. www.countyhealthrankings.org.

Cram, Peter, Laura A. Hatfield, Pieter Bakx et al. "Variation in Revascularisation Use and Outcomes of Patients in Hospital with Acute Myocardial Infarction across Six High Income Countries: Cross Sectional Cohort Study." *BMJ* 377, no. 8336 (2022): e069164. https://doi.org/10.1136/bmj-2021-069164.

Cutler, David M., and Zirui Song. "The New Role of Private Investment in Health Care Delivery." *JAMA Health Forum* 5, no. 2 (2024): e240164. http://doi.org/10.1001/jamahealthforum.2024.0164.

Daly, Rich. "4 Bipartisan Healthcare Policy Changes are Likely in 2025." *Healthcare Financial Management Association*, September 30, 2024. www.hfma.org.

Das, Jishnu, Liana Woskie, Ruma Rajbhandari, Kamran Abbasi, and Ashish Jha. "Rethinking Assumptions about Delivery of Healthcare: Implications for Universal Health Coverage." *BMJ* 361, no. 8154 (2018): k1716. https://doi.org/10.1136/bmj.k1716.

Davies, Gawaine Powell, David Perkins, Julie McDonald, and Anna Williams. "Integrated Primary Health Care in Australia." *International Journal of Integrated Care* 9, no. 4 (2009): e95. http://doi.org/10.5334/ijic.328.

Democratic National Committee. "Achieving Universal, Affordable, Quality Health Care." Accessed December 24, 2024. https://democrats.org.

Dobbels, Fabienne, Rita Van Damme-Lombaert, Johan Vanhaecke, and Sabina De Geest. "Growing Pains: Non-Adherence with the Immunosuppressive Regimen in Adolescent Transplant Recipients." *Pediatric Transplantation* 9, no. 3 (2005): 381–390. https://doi.org/10.1111/j.1399-3046.2005.00356.x.

Domestic Policy Council. *The U.S. Playbook to Address Social Determinants of Health*. Last modified November 2023. www.whitehouse.gov.

Donabedian, Avedis. "Evaluating the Quality of Medical Care." *The Milbank Quarterly* 83, no. 4 (2005): 691–729. https://doi.org/10.1111/j.1468-0009.2005.00397.x.

Duan, Rui-Rui, Ke Hao, and Ting Yang. "Air Pollution and Chronic Obstructive Pulmonary Disease." *Chronic Diseases and Translational Medicine* 6, no. 4 (2020): 260–269. http://doi.org/10.1016/j.cdtm.2020.05.004.

Durrance-Bagale, Anna, Manar Marzouk, Lam Sze Tung et al. "Community Engagement in Health Systems Interventions and Research in Conflict-Affected Countries: A Scoping Review of Approaches." *Global Health Action* 15, no. 1 (2022): 2074131. http://doi.org/10.1080/16549716.2022.2074131.

Dwyer, Devin. "Memo Reveals Only 6 People Signed Up for Obamacare on First Day." *ABC News*, November 1, 2013. https://abcnews.go.com.

Eldridge, Noel, Yun Wang, Mark Metersky et al. "Trends in Adverse Event Rates in Hospitalized Patients, 2010–2019." *JAMA* 328, no. 2 (2022): 173–183. http://doi.org/10.1001/jama.2022.9600.

Ellis, Louise A., Yvonne Tran, Chiara Pomare et al. "Hospital Organizational Change: The Importance of Teamwork Culture, Communication, and Change Readiness." *Frontiers Public Health* 11 (2023): 1–9. http://doi.org/10.3389/fpubh.2023.1089252.

Eozenou, Patrick Hoang-Vu, Sven Neelsen, and Ana Florina Pirlea. "Universal Health Coverage as a Sustainable Development Goal." *World Bank*, January 18, 2023. https://datatopics.worldbank.org.

European Commission. *Health and Well-Being*. Last modified November 28, 2023. https://national-policies.eacea.ec.europa.eu.

Eurostat. "Unmet Health Care Needs Statistics." Accessed December 2, 2024. https://ec.europa.eu.

Federal Communications Commission. *Advancing Broadband Connectivity as a Social Determinant of Health*. Last modified February 7, 2022. www.fcc.gov.

Finkel, Eli J., Christopher A. Bail, Mina Cikara et al. "Political Sectarianism in America." *Science* 370, no. 6516 (2020): 533–536. https://doi.org/10.1126/science.abe1715.

Fleary, Sasha A., and Reynolette Ettienne. "Social Disparities in Health Literacy in the United States." *Health Literacy Research and Practice* 3, no. 1 (2019): e47–e52. https://doi.org/10.3928/24748307-20190131-01.

Freed, Meredith, Jeannie Fuglesten Biniek, Anthony Damico, and Tricia Neuman. "Medicare Advantage in 2024: Enrollment Update and Key Trends." *KFF*, August 8, 2024. www.kff.org.

Frelle-Petersen, Claus, Andreas Hein, and Mathias Christiansen. "The Nordic Social Welfare Model: Lessons for Reform." *Deloitte*, 2020. https://www.deloitte.com/us/en.html.

Gallup. "West Health-Gallup Healthcare Affordability and Value Indexes 2021–2024 Report." Accessed December 7, 2024. www.gallup.com.

GBD 2019 Healthcare Access and Quality Collaborators. "Assessing Performance of the Healthcare Access and Quality Index, Overall and by Select Age Groups, for 204 Countries and Territories, 1990–2019: A Systematic Analysis from the Global Burden of Disease Study 2019." *Lancet Glob Health* 10, no. 12 (2022): e1715–e1743. https://doi.org/10.1016/dS2214-109X(22)00429-6.

Gillespie, James J., and Gregory J. Privitera. "Bringing Patient Incentives into the Bundled Payments Model: Making Reimbursement More Patient-Centric Financially." *International Journal of Healthcare Management* 12, no. 3 (2019): 197–206. http://doi.org/10.1080/20479700.2018.1425276.

Gillespie, James J., and Gregory J. Privitera. *Patient-Centric Analytics in Health Care: Driving Value in Clinical Settings and Psychological Practice*. Lexington Books, 2018.

Gu, Kristine D., Katherine C. Faulknerf, and Anne N. Thorndike. "Housing Instability and Cardiometabolic Health in the United States: A Narrative Review of the Literature." *BMC Public Health* 23 (2023): 931. https://doi.org/10.1186/s12889-023-15875-6.

Guth, Madeline, Rachel Garfield, and Robin Rudowitz. "The Effects of Medicaid Expansion under the ACA: Studies from January 2014 to January 2020." *KFF*, March 17, 2020. www.kff.org.

Hale, Jessica, Nianyi Hong, Ben Hopkins, and Sean Lyons. Eamon Molloy and the Congressional Budget Office Coverage Team. "Health Insurance Coverage Projections for the US Population and Sources of Coverage, by Age, 2024–34." *Health Affairs* 43, no. 7 (2024): 909–1053. https://doi.org/10.1377/hlthaff.2024.00460.

Harris, Ben, Neil R. Mehrotra, and Eric So. "The Fiscal Frontier: Projecting AI's Long-Term Impact on the US Fiscal Outlook." *Brookings Institution*, October 16, 2024. www.brookings.edu.

HealthCare.gov. *Federally Qualified Health Center (FQHC)*. Accessed December 25, 2024. www.healthcare.gov.

HealthCare.gov. *The Children's Health Insurance Program (CHIP)*. Accessed December 25, 2024. www.healthcare.gov.

Health Research & Educational Trust. "Becoming a Culturally Competent Health Care Organization." *American Hospital Association*, June 2013. www.aha.org.

Health Resources & Services Administration. "About the Health Center Program." Last modified August 2024. https://bphc.hrsa.gov.

Hill, Latoya, Samantha Artiga, and Anthony Damico. "Health Coverage by Race and Ethnicity, 2010–2022." *KFF*, January 11, 2024. www.kff.org.

Hoffman, Kelly M., Sophie Trawalter, Jordan R. Axt, and M. Norman Oliver. "Racial Bias in Pain Assessment and Treatment Recommendations, and False Beliefs about Biological Differences between Blacks and Whites." *Proceedings of the National Academy of Sciences of the United States of America* 113, no. 16 (2016): 4296–4301. https://doi.org/10.1073/pnas.1516047113.

Honavar, Santosh G. "Electronic Medical Records – The Good, the Bad and the Ugly." *Indian Journal of Ophthalmology* 68, no. 3 (2020): 417–418. https://doi.org/10.4103/ijo.IJO_278_20.

Housing First Europe. "Denmark." Accessed December 24, 2024. https://housingfirsteurope.eu.

Human Rights Campaign Foundation. "Healthcare Equality Index 2024." Last modified May 2024. www.hrc.org.

Immad, Laiba. "20 Countries with the Best Healthcare in 2024." *Yahoo Finance*, March 14, 2024. https://finance.yahoo.com.

Independent Healthcare Providers Network. "New Research Shows NHS Challenges Driving Demand for Private Healthcare, Particularly among Younger People." Last modified September 10, 2023. www.ihpn.org.uk.

Institute for Healthcare Improvement. "Patient Safety Essentials Toolkit: Ask Me 3." Last modified May 13, 2019. www.ihi.org.

Institute of Medicine. *Unequal Treatment: Confronting Racial and Ethnic Disparities in Health Care*. National Academies Press, 2003. http://doi.org/10.17226/12875.

Jacobs, Lawrence R., Suzanne Mettler, and Ling Zhu. "The Pathways of Policy Feedback: How Health Reform Influences Political Efficacy and Participation." *Policy Studies Journal* 50, no. 3 (2021): 483–506. https://doi.org/10.1111/psj.12424.

Jain, Sanjula. "2023 Trends Shaping the Health Economy." *Trilliant Health*, September 2023. www.trillianthealth.com.

Jiang, Fei, Yongmei Liu, Junhua Hu, and Xiaohong Chen. "Understanding Health Empowerment from the Perspective of Information Processing: Questionnaire Study." *Journal of Medical Internet Research* 24, no. 1 (2022): e27178. http://doi.org/10.2196/27178.

Jindal, Monique, Krisda H. Chaiyachati, Vicki Fung, Spero M. Manson, and Karoline Mortensen. "Eliminating Health Care Inequities through Strengthening Access to Care." *Health Services Research* 58, no. S3 (2023): 300–310. https://doi.org/10.1111/1475-6773.14202.

Jones, Nicholas, Rachel Marks, Roberto Ramirez, and Merarys Ríos-Vargas. "Improved Race and Ethnicity Measures Reveal U.S. Population Is Much

More Multiracial." *United States Census Bureau*, August 12, 2021. www.census.gov.

Joudyian, Nasrin, Leila Doshmangir, Mahdi Mahdavi, Jafar Sadegh Tabrizi, and Vladimir Sergeevich Gordeev. "Public-Private Partnerships in Primary Health Care: A Scoping Review." *BMC Health Services Research* 21, no. 1 (2021): 4. http://doi.org/10.1186/s12913-020-05979-9.

Kaiser Family Foundation. "Status of State Medicaid Expansion Decisions." Last modified November 12, 2024. www.kff.org.

Kaiser Family Foundation. "Tracking Section 1332 State Innovation Waivers." Last modified November 1, 2020. www.kff.org.

Kamal, Rabah and Cynthia Cox. "How Do Healthcare Prices and Use in the U.S. Compare to Other Countries?" *Peterson-KFF Health System Tracker*, May 8, 2018. www.healthsystemtracker.org.

Katz, Mitchell. "What the US Health Care System Assumes about You." *TED Talk*, Palm Springs, CA, November 2018. Video, 15 min., 50 sec. www.ted.com.

Katz Olson, Laura. "Health Care." In *Guide to State Politics and Policy*. Edited by Richard G. Niemi and Joshua J. Dyck, 392–406. CQ Press, 2013.

Keehan, Sean P., Jacqueline A. Fiore, John A. Poisal et al. "National Health Expenditure Projections, 2022–31: Growth To Stabilize Once the COVID-19 Public Health Emergency Ends." *Health Affairs* 42, no. 7 (2023): 886–898. https://doi.org/10.1377/hlthaff.2023.00403.

Keisler-Starkey, Katherine, and Lisa N. Bunch. "Health Insurance Coverage in the United States: 2023." *U.S. Census Bureau*, September 10, 2024. www.census.gov.

KFF. "Primary Care Health Professional Shortage Areas (HPSAs)." Last modified April 1, 2024. www.kff.org.

Kreuter, Matthew W., Tess Thompson, Amy McQueen, and Rachel Garg. "Addressing Social Needs in Health Care Settings: Evidence, Challenges, and Opportunities for Public Health." *Annual Review of Public Health* 42 (2021): 329–344. https://doi.org/10.1146/annurev-publhealth-090419-102204.

Krist, Alex H., Sebastian T. Tong, Rebecca A. Aycock, and Daniel R. Longo. "Engaging Patients in Decision-Making and Behavior Change to Promote Prevention." *Studies in Health Technology and Informatics* 240 (2017): 284–302. https://pmc.ncbi.nlm.nih.gov.

Lam, Onyi, Brian Broderick, and Skye Toor. "How Far Americans Live from the Closest Hospital Differs by Community Type." *Pew Research Center*, December 12, 2018. www.pewresearch.org.

Landon, Bruce E., Gabe Weinreb, and Asaf Bitton. "Making Sense of New Approaches to Primary Care Delivery: A Typology of Innovations in Primary Care." *NEJM Catalyst*, May 9, 2022. https://catalyst.nejm.org.

Lansing, Amy E., Natalie J. Romero, Elizabeth Siantz et al. "Building Trust: Leadership Reflections on Community Empowerment and Engagement in a Large Urban Initiative." *BMC Public Health* 23, no. 1252 (2023): http://doi.org/10.1186/s12889-023-15860-z.

Legatum Institute. "The Legatum Prosperity Index 2023." Accessed December 16, 2024. www.prosperity.com/rankings.

Lennox, Laura, A. Linwood-Amor, L. Maher, and Julie Reed. "Making Change Last? Exploring the Value of Sustainability Approaches in Healthcare: A Scoping Review." *Health Research Policy and Systems* 18 (2020): 120. https://doi.org/10.1186/s12961-020-00601-0.

Lerman, Amy E., Meredith L. Sadin, and Samuel Trachtman. "Policy Uptake as Political Behavior: Evidence from the Affordable Care Act." *American Political Science Review* 111, no. 4 (2017): 755–770. https://doi.org/10.1017/S0003055417000272.

Levinson, Meira, Alan C. Geller, and Joseph G. Allen. "Health Equity, Schooling Hesitancy, and the Social Determinants of Learning." *Lancet Regional Health – Americas* 2 (2021): 100032. http://doi.org/10.1016/j.lana.2021.100032.

Levitt, Larry. "Increasingly Privatized Public Health Insurance Programs in the US." *JAMA Health Forum* 4, no. 3 (2023): e231012. http://doi.org/10.1001/jamahealthforum.2023.1012.

Lier, Elisabeth J., Marjan de Vries, Eline M. Steggink, Richard P. G. Ten Broek, and Harry van Goor. "Effect Modifiers of Virtual Reality in Pain Management: A Systematic Review and Meta-Regression Analysis." *Pain* 164, no. 8 (2023): 1658–1665. http://doi.org/10.1097/j.pain.0000000000002883.

Longacre, Colleen F., Hannah T. Neprash, Nathan D. Shippee, Todd M. Tuttle, and Beth A. Virnig. "Evaluating Travel Distance to Radiation Facilities among Rural and Urban Breast Cancer Patients in the Medicare Population." *Journal of Rural Health* 36, no. 3 (Summer 2020): 334–346. https://doi.org/10.1111/jrh.12413.

Lopes, Lunna, Alex Montero, Marley Presiado, and Liz Hamel. "Americans' Challenges with Health Care Costs." *KFF*, March 2024. www.kff.org.

Madden, Blake. "5 Notable Trends from Healthcare Spending Projections." *Hospitalogy*, July 13, 2023. https://hospitalogy.com.

Maqbool, Nabihah, Janet Viveiros, and Mindy Ault. "The Impacts of Affordable Housing on Health: A Research Summary." *Center for Housing Policy*, April 2015. https://nhc.org.

Maresso, Anna, Ruth Waitzberg, Florian Tille et al. "Engaging the Private Sector in Delivering Health Care and Goods: Governance Lessons from the COVID-19 Pandemic." *World Health Organization*, November 10, 2023. https://eurohealthobservatory.who.int.

Martin, Danielle, Ashley P. Miller, Amélie Quesnel-Vallée et al. "Canada's Universal Health-Care System: Achieving Its Potential." *Lancet* 391, no. 10131 (2018): 1718–1735. http://doi.org/10.1016/S0140-6736(18)30181-8.

Marzban, Sima, Marziye Najafi, Arjola Agolli, and Ensieh Ashrafi. "Impact of Patient Engagement on Healthcare Quality: A Scoping Review." *Journal of Patient Experience* 9 (2022): 23743735221125439. http://doi.org/10.1177/23743735221125439.

Mattke, Soeren, Michael Seid, and Sai Ma. "Evidence for the Effect of Disease Management: Is $1 Billion a Year a Good Investment?" *American Journal of Managed Care* 13, no. 12 (2007): 670–676. https://pubmed.ncbi.nlm.nih.gov.

Medford-Davis, Laura, Rupal Malani, Chelsea Snipes, and Pieter Du Plessis. "The Physician Shortage Isn't Going Anywhere." *McKinsey & Company*, September 10, 2024. www.mckinsey.com.

Medicaid.gov. *Health Related Social Needs*. Accessed December 25, 2024. www.medicaid.gov.

Medical Group Management Association. "Ambient Technology's Role in the Ongoing AI Revolution in Healthcare." Last modified May 23, 2024. www.mgma.com.

Mental Health America. "Quick Facts and Statistics about Mental Health." Accessed December 2, 2024. https://mhanational.org/mentalhealthfacts.

Merahn, Steven. "Humanizing Healthcare: Simple Strategies to Strengthen Patient-Provider Relationships." *Medical Group Management Association*, January 9, 2020. www.mgma.com.

Montori, Victor M., Merel M. Ruissen, Ian G. Hargraves, Juan P. Brito, and Marleen Kunneman. "Shared Decision-Making as a Method of Care." *BMJ Evidence-Based Medicine* 28, no. 4 (2023): 213–217. https://doi.org/10.1136/bmjebm-2022-112068.

Morgan, Rosemary, Tim Ensor, and Hugh Waters. "Performance of Private Sector Health Care: Implications for Universal Health Coverage." *Lancet* 388, no. 10044 (2016): 606–612. http://doi.org/10.1016/S0140-6736(16)00343-3.

Mousa, Tamara Yousef, Daniel Remley, and Ginny Lane. "Editorial: Food Systems, Food Insecurity, and Racial and Ethnic Health Disparities." *Frontiers in Sustainable Food Systems* 7 (April 26, 2023): 1183242. https://doi.org/10.3389/fsufs.2023.1183242.

National Center for Health Statistics. *U.S. Overdose Deaths Decrease in 2023, First Time Since 2018*. 2024. www.cdc.gov.

National Center for Health Statistics. *U.S. Uninsured Rate Dropped 18% during Pandemic*. Last modified May 16, 2023. www.cdc.gov.

National Committee for Quality Assurance (NCQA). "Health Equity and Social Determinants of Health in HEDIS: Data for Measurement." Last modified June 2021. www.ncqa.org.

National Health Service Corps. *Mission, Work, and Impact*. Last modified November 2024. https://nhsc.hrsa.gov/about-us.

National Institute on Drug Abuse. *Drug Overdose Deaths: Facts and Figures*. Last modified August 21, 2024. https://nida.nih.gov.

Ndugga, Nambi, Drishti Pillai, and Samantha Artiga. "Disparities in Health and Health Care: 5 Key Questions and Answers." *KFF*, August 14, 2024. www.kff.org.

Njoku, Anuli, Marian Evans, Lillian Nimo-Sefah, and Jonell Bailey. "Listen to the Whispers before They Become Screams: Addressing Black Maternal Morbidity and Mortality in the United States." *Healthcare* 11, no. 3 (2023): 438. https://doi.org/10.3390/healthcare11030438.

Oberlander, Jonathan. "Polarization, Partisanship, and Health in the United States." *Journal of Health Politics, Policy and Law* 49, no. 3 (2024): 329–350. https://doi.org/10.1215/03616878-11075609.

Office of Disease Prevention and Health Promotion. *Food Is Medicine: A Project to Unify and Advance Collective Action.* Last modified September 29, 2024. https://odphp.health.gov.

Office of Disease Prevention and Health Promotion. *Healthy People 2030.* Accessed December 20, 2024. https://odphp.health.gov.

Organisation for Economic Co-operation and Development (OECD). "OECD Health Statistics." Accessed December 5, 2024. https://data-explorer.oecd.org/.

Organizing Committee for Assessing Meaningful Community Engagement in Health & Health Care Programs & Policies. "Assessing Meaningful Community Engagement: A Conceptual Model to Advance Health Equity through Transformed Systems for Health." *National Academy of Medicine*, February 14, 2022. https://doi.org/10.31478/202202c.

Padilla, Christina M. and Dana Thomson. "Nearly 1 Million More Children Were in Poverty in 2023 than 2022, Despite Economic Growth." *Child Trends*, September 10, 2024. www.childtrends.org.

Papanicolas, Irene, Liana R. Woskie, and Ashish K. Jha. "Health Care Spending in the United States and Other High-Income Countries." *JAMA* 319, no. 10 (2018): 1024–1039. https://doi.org/10.1001/jama.2018.1150.

Parast, Layla, Megan Mathews, Steven Martino et al. "Racial/Ethnic Differences in Emergency Department Utilization and Experience." *Journal of General Internal Medicine* 37, no. 1 (2021): 49–56. https://doi.org/10.1007/s11606-021-06738-0.

Pennic, Fred. "Healthcare Deserts: 80% of U.S. Lacks Adequate Access to Healthcare." *HIT Consultant*, September 10, 2021. https://hitconsultant.net.

Physicians for a National Health Program. "Republican and Democratic Platforms on Health Care." Accessed December 24, 2024. https://pnhp.org.

Pifer, Rebecca. "Healthcare Lobbying Rose 70% over Past Two Decades." *Healthcare Dive*, October 31, 2022. www.healthcaredive.com.

Plescia, Marcus, Claire Hannan, and Jessica Baggett. "A Pandemic Success Story: Distribution and Administration of COVID-19 Vaccines." *Journal of Public Health Management and Practice* 28, no. 6 (2022): 749–750. http://doi.org/10.1097/PHH.0000000000001651.

Raday, Sophia, Alexandra Chan, and Nima Krodel. "Healthy Outcomes Initiative Report and Resources." *Nonprofit Finance Fund*, 2024. https://nff.org.

Radley, David C., Arnav Shah, Sara R. Collins, Neil R. Powe, and Laurie C. Zephyrin. "Advancing Racial Equity in U.S. Health Care: The Commonwealth Fund 2024 State Health Disparities Report." *Commonwealth Fund*, April 18, 2024. www.commonwealthfund.org.

Ranabhat, Chhabi Lal, Shambhu Prasad Acharya, Chiranjivi Adhikari, and Chun-Bae Kim. "Universal Health Coverage Evolution, Ongoing Trend, and Future Challenge: A Conceptual and Historical Policy Review." *Frontiers Public Health* 11 (2023): https://doi.org/10.3389/fpubh.2023.1041459.

Rodrigues, Nuno J. P. "Public–Private Partnerships Model Applied to Hospitals–A Critical Review." *Healthcare (Basel, Switzerland)* 11, no. 12 (2023): 1723. http://doi.org/10.3390/healthcare11121723.

Rovner, Julie. "Congress and the Executive Branch and Health Policy." *KFF*, July 2024. www.kff.org.

Sahni, Nikhil R., Prakriti Mishra, Brandon Carrus, and David M. Cutler. "Administrative Simplification: How to Save a Quarter-Trillion Dollars in US Healthcare." *McKinsey & Company*, October 20, 2021. www.mckinsey.com.

Sarasohn-Kahn, Jane. "In the Past Ten Years, Workers' Health Insurance Premiums Have Grown Much Faster than Wages." *Health Populi*, October 9, 2020. www.healthpopuli.com.

Savoy, Margot, Colleen Hazlett-O'Brien, and Jamie Rapacciuolo. "The Role of Primary Care Physicians in Managing Chronic Disease." *Dela J Public Health* 3, no. 1 (2017): 86–93. https://pmc.ncbi.nlm.nih.gov.

Schpero, William L., Nancy E. Morden, Thomas D. Sequist et al. "For Selected Services, Blacks and Hispanics More Likely to Receive Low-Value Care than Whites." *Health Affairs* 36, no. 6 (2017): 1065–1069. https://doi.org/10.1377/hlthaff.2016.1416.

Schpero, William L., Thomas Wiener, Samuel Carter, and Paula Chatterjee. "Lobbying Expenditures in the US Health Care Sector, 2000–2020." *JAMA Health Forum* 3, no. 10 (2022): e223801. http://doi.org/10.1001/jamahealthforum.2022.3801.

Shegaze Shimbre, Mulugeta, and Abayneh Tunje Tanga. "Perspective Chapter: The Importance of Collaborative Care in Community Health Settings." In *Current Trends in Community Health Models [Working Title]*. Edited by Marco Bassanello, Xin-Nong Li, and Ruggero Geppini. IntechOpen, 2024. http://doi.org/10.5772/intechopen.115212.

Siegrist, Johannes. "Health Inequalities: The Role of Work and Employment." *European Journal of Public Health* 30, no. 4 (2020): 620. https://doi.org/10.1093/eurpub/ckaa006.

Sinaiko, Anna D., Elizabeth Bambury, and Alyna T. Chien. "Consumer Choice in U.S. Health Care: Using Insights from the Past to Inform the Way Forward." *Commonwealth Fund*, November 30, 2021. www.commonwealthfund.org.

Smith, Laura Barrie, Michael Karpman, Dulce Gonzalez, and Sarah Morriss. "More than One in Five Adults with Limited Public Transit Access Forgo Health Care Because of Transportation Barriers." *Robert Wood Johnson Foundation*, April 26, 2023. www.rwjf.org.

Special Olympics Health. "What Is Inclusive Health." Accessed December 26, 2024. https://inclusivehealth.specialolympics.org.

Stenberg, Karin, Odd Hanssen, Tessa Tan-Torres Edejer et al. "Financing Transformative Health Systems towards Achievement of the Health Sustainable Development Goals: A Model for Projected Resource Needs in 67 Low-Income and Middle-Income Countries." *Lancet Global Health* 5, no. 9 (2017): e875–e887. https://doi.org/10.1016/S2214-109X(17)30263-2.

Sutton, Madeline Y., Ngozi F. Anachebe, Regina Lee, and Heather Skanes. "Racial and Ethnic Disparities in Reproductive Health Services and Outcomes, 2020." *Obstetrics and Gynecology* 137, no. 2 (2021): 225–233. https://doi.org/10.1097/AOG.0000000000004224.

Takeshita, Junko, Shiyu Wang, Alison W. Loren et al. "Association of Racial/Ethnic and Gender Concordance between Patients and Physicians with Patient Experience Ratings." *JAMA Network Open* 3, no. 11 (2020): e2024583. http://doi.org/10.1001/jamanetworkopen.2020.24583.

Thomas, Alexander, Javier Valero-Elizondo, Rohan Khera et al. "Forgone Medical Care Associated with Increased Health Care Costs among the U.S. Heart Failure Population." *Science Direct* 9, no. 10 (2021): 710–719. https://doi.org/10.1016/j.jchf.2021.05.010.

Thomas Craig, Kelly Jean, Nicole Fusco, Thrudur Gunnarsdottir et al. "Leveraging Data and Digital Health Technologies to Assess and Impact Social Determinants of Health (SDoH)." *Online Journal of Public Health Informatics* 13, no. 3 (2021): e62617. http://doi.org/10.5210/ojphi.v13i3.11081.

Totz, Rachael. "Expanding Access to Food as Medicine." *Regulatory Review*, December 4, 2024. www.theregreview.org.

Trachtman, Samuel. "Polarization, Participation, and Premiums: How Political Behavior Helps Explain Where the ACA Works, and Where It Doesn't." *Journal of Health Politics, Policy and Law* 44, no. 6 (2019): 855–884. https://doi.org/10.1215/03616878-7785787.

Truveta Research. "SDOH Factors Like Housing and Financial Stability Are Key to Medication Adherence." October 17, 2023. www.truveta.com.

United States Census Bureau. *2023 National Population Projections Tables: Main Series*. 2023. www.census.gov.

United States Census Bureau. *By 2030, All Baby Boomers Will Be Age 65 or Older*. December 10, 2019. www.census.gov.

Urgent Care Association. "The Essential Nature of Urgent Care in the Healthcare Ecosystem Post-COVID-19." *Urgent Care Association*, August 2023. https://urgentcareassociation.org.

U.S. Bureau of Labor Statistics. *Occupational Employment and Wages, May 2023*. April 3, 2024. www.bls.gov.

U.S. Centers for Disease Control and Prevention. *CDC's Health Literacy Action Plan*. Last modified October 16, 2024. www.cdc.gov.

U.S. Centers for Disease Control and Prevention. *Global Water, Sanitation and Hygiene*. Last modified November 6, 2024. www.cdc.gov.

U.S. Centers for Disease Control and Prevention. *Patient-Centered Medical Home (PCMH) Model*. Last modified May 15, 2024. www.cdc.gov.

U.S. Centers for Disease Control and Prevention. *Social Determinants of Health*. Last modified February 7, 2024. www.cdc.gov.

U.S. Centers for Disease Control and Prevention. *Social Determinants of Health (SDOH)*. Last modified January 17, 2024. www.cdc.gov.

U.S. Centers for Disease Control and Prevention. *Socioeconomic factors*. Last modified September 1, 2023. www.cdc.gov.

U.S. Centers for Medicare & Medicaid Services. *The Mental Health Parity and Addiction Equity Act (MHPAEA)*. Accessed December 25, 2024. www.cms.gov.

U.S. Department of Agriculture. *Broadband*. Accessed December 6, 2024. www.usda.gov/broadband.

U.S. Department of Agriculture. *ERS Charts of Note*. September 25, 2024. www.ers.usda.gov.

U.S. Department of Health and Human Services. *Advancing Health Equity at Every Point of Contact*. Accessed December 26, 2024. https://thinkculturalhealth.hhs.gov.

U.S. Department of Health and Human Services. "COVID-19 Vaccines." Last modified March 13, 2024. www.hhs.gov.

U.S. Department of Health and Human Services. *Healthy People 2030*. Accessed December 7, 2024. https://odphp.health.gov.

U.S. Department of Health and Human Services. *Healthy People 2030: Building a Healthier Future for All*. Accessed December 11, 2024. https://odphp.health.gov.

U.S. Department of Health and Human Services. *Social Determinants of Health*. Accessed December 11, 2024. https://odphp.health.gov.

U.S. Department of State. *Patient Bill of Rights and Responsibilities*. Accessed December 25, 2024. www.state.gov.

U.S. Environmental Protection Agency. *Particle Pollution and Respiratory Effects*. Last modified June 20, 2024. www.epa.gov.

U.S. Food and Drug Administration. "Laws, Regulations, Policies and Procedures for Drug Applications." Last modified December 4, 2014. www.fda.gov.

US Preventive Services Task Force. "Collaboration and Shared Decision-Making between Patients and Clinicians in Preventive Health Care Decisions and US Preventive Services Task Force Recommendations." *JAMA* 327, no. 12 (2022): 1171–1176. http://doi.org/10.1001/jama.2022.3267.

Van Bavel, Jay J., Shana Kushner Gadarian, Eric Knowles, and Kai Ruggeri. "Political Polarization and Health." *Nature Medicine* 30 (2024): 3085–3093. https://doi.org/10.1038/s41591-024-03307-w.

Villas-Boas, Sofia, Scott Kaplan, Justin S. White, and Renee Y. Hsia. "Patterns of US Mental Health–Related Emergency Department Visits during the COVID-19 Pandemic." *JAMA Network Open* 6, no. 7 (2023): e2322720. http://doi.org/10.1001/jamanetworkopen.2023.22720.

Vlaev, Ivo, Dominic King, Ara Darzi, and Paul Dolan. "Changing Health Behaviors Using Financial Incentives: A Review from Behavioral Economics." *BMC Public Health* 19, no. 1059 (2019): 1059. https://doi.org/10.1186/s12889-019-7407-8.

Wager, Emma, and Cynthia Cox. "International Comparison of Health Systems." *KFF*, May 28, 2024. www.kff.org.

Wager, Emma, Imani Telesford, Shameek Rakshit, Nisha Kurani, and Cynthia Cox. "How Does the Quality of the U.S. Health System Compare to Other Countries?" *Peterson-KFF Health System Tracker*, October 9, 2024. www.healthsystemtracker.org.

Wager, Emma, Matthew McGough, Shameek Rakshit, Krutika Amin, and Cynthia Cox. "How Does Health Spending in the U.S. Compare to Other Countries?" *Petersson-KFF Health System Tracker*. January 2024. www.healthsystemtracker.org.
Wang, Yiting, Wenhui Hou, Xiaokang Wang, Hongyu Zhang, and Jianqiang Wang. "Bad to All? A Novel Way to Analyze the Effects of Fee-for-Service on Multiple Grades Hospitals Operation Outcomes." *International Journal of Environmental Research and Public Health* 18, no. 23: (2021): 12723. http://doi.org/10.3390/ijerph182312723.
Wang, Ming-Jye, and Yi-Ting Lo. "Strategies for Improving the Utilization of Preventive Care Services: Application of Importance–Performance Gap Analysis Method." *International Journal of Environmental Research and Public Health* 19, no. 20 (2022): 13195. https://doi.org/10.3390/ijerph192013195.
Washburn, Kaitlin. "Nearly 43,000 People Died from Gun Violence in 2023: How to Tell the Story." *Association of Health Care Journalists*, February 14, 2024. https://healthjournalism.org.
Weiss, Daniel J., Andy Nelson, Carlos A. Vargas-Ruiz et al. "Global Maps of Travel Time to Healthcare Facilities." *Nature Medicine* 26 (2020): 1835–1838. https://doi.org/10.1038/s41591-020-1059-1.
White House. *FACT SHEET: The Congressional Republican Agenda: Repealing the Affordable Care Act and Slashing Medicaid*. Last modified February 28, 2023. www.whitehouse.gov.
World Economic Forum. "Healthcare Pays the Highest Price of Any Sector for Cyberattacks – That's Why Cyber Resilience Is Key." Last modified February 1, 2024. www.weforum.org.
World Health Organization. "Consensus Statement: Role of Policy-Makers and Health Care Leaders in Implementation of the Global Patient Safety Action Plan 2021–2030." Last modified February 24, 2022. https://iris.who.int.
World Health Organization. "Patient Engagement: Technical Series on Safer Primary Care." Last modified 2016. https://iris.who.int.
World Health Organization. "Quality of Care." Accessed August 21, 2024. www.who.int.
World Health Organization. "Universal Health Coverage." Accessed December 16, 2024. www.who.int.
World Health Organization. "WHO Estimates Cost of Reaching Global Health Targets by 2030." Last modified July 17, 2017. www.who.int.
World Population Review. "Healthiest Countries 2024." Accessed December 26, 2024. https://worldpopulationreview.com.
World Population Review. "Most Racially Diverse Countries 2024." Accessed July 20, 2024. https://worldpopulationreview.com.
Worrall, Ashley. "What Is Patient Experience and Why Is It Important in Healthcare?" *Feedtrail*, November 6, 2024. www.feedtrail.com.
Wright, Jenna and Jeanna Holtz. "Essential Packages of Health Services in 24 Countries: Findings from a Cross-Country Analysis." *Health Finance and Governance Project*, June 2017. www.hfgproject.org.

Wu, Jingxian, Yongmei Yang, Ting Sun, and Sucen He. "Inequalities in Unmet Health Care Needs under Universal Health Insurance Coverage in China." *Health Economics Review* 14, no. 2 (2024): https://doi.org/10.1186/s13561-023-00473-4.

Yabroff, K. Robin, Joanna F. Doran, Jingxuan Zhao et al. "Cancer Diagnosis and Treatment in Working-Age Adults: Implications for Employment, Health Insurance Coverage, and Financial Hardship in the United States." *American Cancer Society* 74, no. 4 (2024): 341–358. https://doi.org/10.3322/caac.21837.

Younas, Ahtisham, Sharoon Shahzad, Clara Isabel Tejada-Garrido, Esther Nyangate Monari, and Angela Durante. "Sociocultural and Patient-Health Care Professional Related Factors Influencing Self-Management of Multiethnic Patients with Multimorbidities: A Thematic Synthesis." *PLOS Global Public Health* 3, no. 9 (2023): e0002132. https://doi.org/10.1371/journal.pgph.0002132.

Zajacova, Anna, and Elizabeth M. Lawrence. "The Relationship between Education and Health: Reducing Disparities through a Contextual Approach." *Annual Review of Public Health* 39 (2018): 273–289. https://doi.org/10.1146/annurev-publhealth-031816-044628.

Zorthian, Julia. "Why It's Important to 'Meet People Where They Are' When Improving U.S. Healthcare." *TIME*, April 24, 2024. https://time.com.

Index

6 Ps framework for health care
  alignment of interests across, 164
  introduction and overview, x, 8, 12–13
  patients, 13–14
  payers, 18–19
  pharmaceutical companies, 17–18
  pharmacies, 16–17
  policy makers, 14–15
  providers, 15–16
21st Century Cures Act, 81
340B Drug Pricing Program, 129

access and accessibility, *see also* equity; inclusive health care
  geographical accessibility, 9, 44, 45–46, 48–49, 56, 121, 123–124
  Health Professional Shortage Areas (HPSAs), 44
  Health care Access and Quality Index (HAQ), 8–9
  importance of, 29
  language barriers, 46, 109
  and medication adherence, 108
  as necessary but not sufficient for health equity, 102, 107–108, 112
  other measures of, 9–10
  and primary care physicians (PCPs), 30, 120, 141–142
Accountable Care Organization (ACO), 161
Accountable Health Communities (AHC) model, 142
Accountable Health Communities Model, 110
adverse events, US performance in, 33
advocacy
  and Older Americans Act (OAA), 144
  patient advocacy groups, 13, 153–155
  payers, 19
  pharmaceutical companies, 18
  pharmacies, 16
  physicians, 157
  policy makers, 14

  and social determinants of health (SDOH) framework, 106–107
  training in, 159
affordability, 29–30, 39, 41–44, 102, *see also* costs and spending
Affordable Care Act (ACA)
  Accountable Health Communities Model, 110
  vs. American Health Care Act (AHCA), x, 126–128
  Community Health Center Fund, 81
  costs under, 90–93
  and discrimination prohibition, 139
  and disincentivizing employment, 94
  enrollment on insurance exchange, 89, 92–93
  goals and launch, 88–89, 117–118
  and health insurance complexity, 89–90
  health insurance provisions, 77, 88, 89
  impact on health care marketplace, 90
  key provisions, 144
  and Medicaid expansion, 89, 90–91, 110, 129
  National Prevention Council and Strategy, 110
  and partisanship, 77, 141
  and social determinants of health (SDOH), 110
  uneven implementation, 149
Affordable Drug Pricing Act, 81
age
  and health outcomes, 32
  support for aging populations, 143–144
ageism, 32
Agency for Health care Research and Quality (AHRQ), 120
air quality, and health outcomes, 108
American Diabetes Association, 66
American Health Care Act (AHCA), x, 126–128
American Heart Association, 66
American Red Cross, 66
artificial intelligence (AI), 52, 55, 67, 84, 97–100
Ask Me 3 program, 13
assumptions, of health care system, 109
augmented and virtual reality (AR and VR), 85

189

Index

Australia
  health promotion campaigns, 111
  health care model and performance, 25, 26, 124
  integration of social services and health care, 150
Austria, 29
autonomy
  and Community-Engaged Health care (CEH), 155
  and incentive misalignment between patients, providers, and payers, 41

Beveridge model (health care system), xi, 5, 6, 61
Bismarck model (health care system), xi, 5, 6–7, 61–62
blockchain technology, 99
Bloomberg Global Health Index, 21
Bloomberg Health Index, 124–125
brain–computer interfaces (BCIs), 85
broadband access, 46, 48, see also telehealth

Canada, 25, 62, 150
care process, US performance in, 32–33
Carnegie, Dale, *How to Win Friends and Influence People*, 101–102
Centers for Disease Control and Prevention (CDC), 123, 156
Centers for Medicare & Medicaid Services (CMS), 142, 145
child poverty, 36
Children's Health Insurance Program (CHIP), 65, 81, 141
China, 62
citizenship status, and health disparities, 32
Community Engagement Alliance, 123
community forums and decision-making, 79, 82, 155, 158
community health centers (CHCs), 81, 110, 130, 140
  Federally Qualified Health Centers (FQHCs), 48–49, 142–143
community health workers (CHWs), 51, 155
community leader – health care organization (HCO) collaboration, 157–160, 162–163
community resources, leveraging, 158–159
Community-Engaged Health care (CEH), x, 153–155
comparisons and trends (in the United States)
  aging population, 143
  federal government spending on health insurance, 71
  health care spending relative to GDP, 27, 90
  hospital closures, 46
  life expectancy, 94, 95
  lobbying, 38
  maternal and infant mortality, 36
  partisanship prevalence, 72
  private vs. public insurance administrative costs, 42
  urgent care clinics, 82
comparisons and trends (methods)
  benchmarking analysis, 25
  constrained optimization modeling, 25
  trendline analysis, 25
comparisons and trends (United States and other countries)
  advanced technology uptake, 34
  care process, 32–33
  drug costs, 64
  ethnic diversity and health outcomes, xi, 20, 21
  health care price per unit, 28
  health care spending per capita, 26
  life expectancy, 36, 125
  long-term care spending per capita, 33
  maternal and infant mortality, 36
  number of physicians per 1,000 people, 30
  overall health care performance, 25–26, 62, 124–125, 141
  preventive care spending, 33
  social services vs. health services investment, 112–113
  unmet health care needs, 29
contracting-out and contracting-in services, 66
copays (in health insurance), 41–42
costs and spending, see also affordability; health insurance
  and advanced technologies, 34
  cost efficiencies of universal health care, 125
  data security violations, 84
  debt problems, 43, 71–72
  drug prices, 17, 81, 128, 129
  federal government spending on health insurance, 71
  hospital vs. ambulatory care, 33
  impact of artificial intelligence (AI), 97, 98
  and incentive misalignment between patients, providers, and payers, 41, 96–97
  as lead driver of federal government spending, 39, 73
  and life expectancy, x, 26
  measurement, xi, 10
  payers in 6 Ps framework, 18–19
  prescription drugs and equipment, costs per capita, 28, 64
  preventive care expenditure, 33, 96–97
  price per unit, 28–29, 64
  pricing model transparency, 82, 93, 149–150
  social services investment, 112–113
  spending per capita, country comparisons, 26
  spending relative to GDP, 27, 90

and utilization, 27–28
and whole being model, 137
COVID-19 pandemic
  and ethnicity, access, and outcome disparities, 30, 120
  excess deaths (US), 36
  expanded role of pharmacies, 156
  impact on health care workers, 45
  Medicaid and Children's Health Insurance Program (CHIP), 120
  and mental health, 32
  mobile medical services, 49
  partisanship, 77
  public–private partnerships (PPPs), 56–57
  vaccine distribution, 4, 156
cultural competency, 144–145
cultural/political determinants of health, 76–77, 105
Czech Republic
  health care model, 6
  unmet health care needs, 29

data and digital technology
  analytics for tailored interventions, 137–138, 159
  artificial intelligence (AI), 52, 55, 67, 84, 97–100
  augmented and virtual reality (AR and VR), 85
  brain–computer interfaces (BCIs), 85
  data sharing and standards, 67, 82, 84, 159
  and decision-making, 82
  and Healthy People 2030 framework, x, 118, 119
  importance for universal health care, 52
  internet (broadband) access, 46, 48
  Internet of Medical Things (IoMT), 84
  predictive analytics, 83–84
  remote patient monitoring (RPM), 85
  routine task automation, 85, 98–99
  security issues, 84
debt problems, 43, 71–72
deductibles (in health insurance), x, 41–42, 43, 64, 92
defensive medicine, 64, 96
Denmark
  health care model and performance, 131
  integration of social determinants into health care policies, 131–132
diagnostic care, impact of artificial intelligence (AI), 98, 99
discrimination, 30, 32, 120
  antidiscrimination legislation, 139
disruptive innovation, 66–67

diversity
  Fractionalization Index, 20
  of health care workforce, 141–142, 146
  national ethnic diversity vs. health, xi, 19–20, 21
  and patient-centered approach, 20–22
Donabedian model (health care quality), x, 8, 9
drugs
  affordability, 29
  costs per capita, 28, 64
  development, 17, 81
  direct-to-consumer supply, 83
  legal definitions, 114
  medication management, 16
  over-the-counter medicines, 41, 114
  pricing, 17, 81, 128, 129
  supply chain management, 17
  under-prescribing for Black and Hispanic patients, 120

early childhood development policies, 110
education (of public/patients)
  access to/levels of, and health outcomes, 122, 132
  community leader training, 159
  and depolarized decision-making, 83
  and empowerment, 51, 83, 157, 159
  health literacy, 51, 139, 159
  integrative education/health policies, 132, 158
emergency departments (EDs)
  affordability, 42
  and after-hour care, 30
  educating the public about, 42
  and mental health care, 80
  mobile solutions, 49
  over-reliance on by Black and Hispanic patients, 120
empathy, 146, 147, 148–149
employer-provided health insurance
  and Bismarck model, 6
  costs and coverage issues, x, 43, 91–92
  disadvantages, 71
  eligibility, 43
  prevalence in United States, 34
  tax benefits, 63
  universal coverage and, 35
empowerment, 51
environmental conditions, and health outcomes, 108
equality, *see also* inequalities
  vs. equity and justice, 3–4
equity, *see also* inequities (disparities)
  and accessibility (as necessary but not sufficient), 102, 107–108, 112

equity (cont.)
  and Community-Engaged Health care (CEH), 155
  and COVID-19 vaccine distribution, 4
  definition and underlying concepts, 103
  vs. equality and justice, 3–4
  and health-related social needs (HRSN), 47–48
  in health care access, 9–10
  inclusive health care. *see* inclusive health care
  and legislation (in general), 139
  and meeting people where they are, 102–103, 108, 118, 123–124, 155, 156–157, 159–160
  and public–private partnerships (PPPs), 65–66, 128–129
  and social determinants of health (SDOH), 102, *see* social determinants of health (SDOH)
  social programs for, 65
  and universal health care, 125
Essential Packages of Health Services (EPHS), 56
ethnicity and race
  and health disparities, x, 30, 31, 36, 113, 119–121
  and health insurance, 119–120, 121
  and health care debt, 43
  national ethnic diversity and health outcomes, xi, 20, 21
excess (in health insurance), *see* deductibles (in health insurance)

Federally Qualified Health Centers (FQHCs), 48–49, 142–143
fee-for-service (FFS) payment model, 96, 160
financial incentives, *see also* payment models
  challenges and opportunities, 163
  for patients, x, 161–163
  pay for performance, 96, 160–161
food
  food deserts, 47, 130
  food insecurity, 108, 109, 110, 122, 124
  as medicine, 114–115
Food and Drug Administration (FDA), 114
Fractionalization Index (of ethnic diversity), 20
France
  health care model, 6, 62
  overall health care performance (comparative data), 25
fraud, 91, 99

gender/sexual identity and orientation
  and health disparities, 32
  and health care debt, 43
gene therapies, 85–86

geographical accessibility, 9, 44, 45–46, 48–49, 56, 121, 123–124
Germany
  health care model and performance, 6, 25, 29, 35, 62, 150
  unmet health care needs, 29
global health initiatives, 17
good target incentives, x, 162, *see also* financial incentives

Health Center Program, 140, *see also* community health centers (CHCs)
health equity, *see* equity
health insurance, *see also* uninsured/under-insured persons
  administrative costs, 42, 52, 64, 71, 91
  and Bismarck model, xi, 5, 6–7, 61–62
  Children's Health Insurance Program (CHIP), 65, 81, 141
  claims processing, 19
  complexities of US system, 29–30, 63–64, 71, 89–90
  copays, 41–42
  deductibles, x, 41–42, 43, 64, 92
  employer-provided. *see* employer-provided health insurance
  and ethnicity, 119–120, 121
  federal government spending on, 71
  fraud, 91
  and health care policy, 18–19, 129
  increase in premiums, x, 91–92
  Medicare. *see* Medicare
  and mental health services, 81, 140–141
  and moral hazard, 94
  National Health Insurance Model, xi, 5, 7, 62
  patient navigators to help with choice, 64
  as a political issue, 73–74, 126–128
  provisions under the Affordable Care Act (ACA), 77, 88, 89, 129
  public vs. private insurance (overview and advantages/disadvantages), 54, 59–60
  and risk pool, 92–94
  and telehealth, 129
  and universal coverage, 35
  upcoding, 97
health literacy, 51, 139, 159, *see also* education (of public/patients)
Health Professional Shortage Areas (HPSAs), 44
Health Savings Accounts (HSAs), 126
Health care Access and Quality Index (HAQ), 8–9
Health care Equality Index (HEI), 143
health care organization (HCO) – community leader collaboration, 157–160, 162–163

health care providers, in 6 Ps framework, 15–16
health care workforce
  community health workers (CHWs), 51, 155
  diversity, 141–142, 146
  impact of COVID-19 on, 45
  mental health practitioner shortages, 45
  nurse shortages, 98
  physicians as advocates, 157
  primary care physician (PCP) shortages, 30, 98
health-related social needs (HRSN), 47–48
Healthy People 2030 (framework), x, 115, 118, 119
housing instability, 47, 94, 101, 105, 108, 113, 121–122, 124, 145
housing interventions, 131, 145, 150
Human Rights Campaign, 143

Iceland, 62, 124
incentive (mis)alignment, x, 39–42, 96–97
incentives, financial. *see* financial incentives
inclusive health care
  definition and importance, 134–135
  steps toward, x, 136, 138–145
  whole being model, x, 135–138, 147–148, 149–151
income, low
  and early childhood development policies, 111
  and health disparities, 30, 45, 49, 59, 108, 109, 112, 113, 121, 122
  and health insurance, *see* uninsured/under-insured persons
  and health insurance, *see* Medicaid
  and health insurance, *see* Children's Health Insurance Program (CHIP)
  and medication adherence, 108
  medication discounts, 129
  and public health interventions, 111
inequalities, *see also* equality
  national ethnic diversity and health outcomes, xi, 20, 21
  social determinants of health, *see* social determinants of health (SDOH)
inequities (disparities), 31, *see also* equity; social determinants of health (SDOH)
  addressing through SDOH-informed policies, x, 105–107
  and built-in assumptions of health care system, 109
  and citizenship status, 32
  closing gaps (key themes), 146–147
  discrimination, *see* discrimination
  and ethnicity, x, 30, 31, 36, 113, 119–121
  and gender/sexual identity and orientation, 32
  and systemic barriers, 119
insurance, *see* health insurance

internet (broadband) access, 46, 48, *see also* telehealth
Internet of Medical Things (IoMT), 84
Israel, 62
Italy, 124, 141

Japan, 6, 62
justice, vs. equality and equity, 3–4

Katz, Mitchell, 109
Korea, 6
  South Korea, 62

language barriers, 46, 109
LGBTQ+-inclusive policies, 143
life expectancy, x, 26, 36, 94, 95
listening to the patient, 147
litigation, fear of, 96
living conditions, and health outcomes, 108
lobbying, 38
long-term care, expenditure, 33

maternal and infant mortality, 36, 45
media and social media
  message framing and depolarization, 79
  motivated reasoning in message interpretation, 74
Medicaid, *see also* income, low
  during COVID-19 pandemic, 120
  expansion, 80–81, 89, 90, 110, 129
  funding and administration, 52, 62–63, 73, 127
  and local health care provision, 49, 51
  and mental health services, 32
Medically Underserved Areas/Populations (MUA/MUPs), 44, *see also* access and accessibility
Medicare, 6, 7, 34, 42, 128
  Medicare Advantage plans, 62–63, 97
medication adherence, 108
medication management, 16
medicine
  drugs, *see* drugs
  legal definitions, 114
  social determinants of health (SDOH) as "medicine," 114–115
Mental Health Parity and Addiction Equity Act (MHPAEA), 81, 140–141
mental health services
  demand for, 79–80
  and health insurance, 81, 140–141
  methods of provision, 80, 140
  practitioner shortages, 45
mental health/illness, 32, 46, 77, 85, 113, 122
mobile clinics, 49, 123–124, 140

moral hazard, 94
motivated reasoning, 74

National Food as Medicine Program Act, 115
National Health Insurance Model (health care system), xi, 5, 7, 62
national health rankings
　Bloomberg Global Health Index, 21
　vs. ethnic diversity, xi, 19–20, 21
National Health Service Corps (NHSC), 141–142
National Institutes of Health (NIH), Community Engagement Alliance, 123
National Prevention Council and Strategy, 110
negative externalities, 39
Netherlands
　health care model, 29, 35
　overall health care performance, 25, 26
　unmet health care needs, 29
New Zealand, 25, 61
Norway, 62, 124
nurses, shortages, 98

Older Americans Act (OAA), 144
opioid abuse disorder, 80, 81, 94
Opioid Crisis Response Act, 81
Organisation for Economic Co-operation and Development (OECD), 70, 112
　2024 health statistics report, 25
out-of-pocket model (health care system), xi, 5, 7, 43–44
over-utilization, 41, 42, 51, 61

participatory model of health care, 153, 155
partisanship and polarization, *see also* politics
　bipartisan health care policymaking, x, 74–75, 78–86, 128–130
　growth and prevalence, 72–73
　impact on health care policymaking, 73–74
　impact on physicians, 73
　and individual health behaviors and outcomes, 76–77
　introduction and definitions, 72
　negative impact of extreme levels on health care policymaking, 74–75, 77–78
　positive impact of healthy levels on health care policymaking, 76
　role of social media, 74
　and trust/risk assessment, 75–76
patient advocacy groups, 13, 153–155
patient feedback, 148
Patient Protection and Affordable Care Act, *see* Affordable Care Act (ACA)
patient-centered care
　in 6 Ps framework, 13–14, 164
　benefits (overview), 153, 164

Community-Engaged Health care (CEH), x, 153–155
　empathy, 146, 147, 148–149
　and ethnic diversity, 20–22
　listening, 147
　participatory model, 153, 155
　Patient-Centered Medical Home (PCMH) model, 139–140
　and reducing polarization, 78, 83
　shift toward, 153
　whole being model, x, 135–138, 147–148, 149–151
patient-reported outcome measures (PROMs), 161
Patients' Bill of Rights, 149
pay for performance (incentive), 96, 160–161
paying for health care, *see* costs and spending
payment models, *see also* financial incentives
　introduction and overview, 18
　pay for performance, 96, 160–161
pharmaceutical companies, in 6 Ps framework, 17–18
pharmacies
　expanded role, 156, 157
　in 6 Ps framework, 16–17
policy makers, in 6 Ps framework, 14–15
politics
　bipartisan health care policymaking, x, 74–75, 78–86, 128–130
　cultural/political determinants of health, 76–77, 105
　Democrat vs. Republican positions on government and health care, 126–128
　health policy/interventions as inherently political, 35, 38, 50–51, 70–71, 73–74, 105, 106, 107, 125–128
　partisanship and polarization, *see* partisanship and polarization
positive externalities, 39
preventive care
　access and outcomes, 51
　and Accountable Care Organization (ACO), 161
　expenditure, 33, 96–97
　and health insurance design, 41–42, 60–60
　opioid abuse prevention, 80, 81
　and patient incentives, 162
　and social determinants of health (SDOH), 113
　and universal health care, 125
primary care
　accessibility, 30, 120, 141–142
　FQHC neighborhood clinics, 48
　mental health services in, 140
　mobile clinics, 49, 123–124, 140

primary care physician (PCP) shortages, 30, 98
school-based health centers (SBHCs), 49
private-sector health care organizations, *see also* public-private partnerships (PPPs)
  attitudes toward, 60–61
  characteristics, 58–59, 66–67
  quality metrics, 65
providers
  in 6 Ps framework, 15–16
  expanding role of, 155–157
public engagement in health care policymaking, 79
public health perspective on health care, 51, 66, 150
public–private partnerships (PPPs)
  contracting-out and contracting-in services, 66
  data sharing, 67
  and disruptive innovation, 66–67
  during COVID-19 pandemic, 56–57
  duties and responsibilities of governments in, 65–66
  guidelines and key considerations, 55–56
  and health equity, 65–66, 128–129
  introduction and definition, 53–54
  in Medicare and Medicaid, 62–63
  potential benefits, 54–55, 57–58, 128–129, 130
  potential drawbacks, 59, 66–67
  toward universal health care, 57–58

quality of health care
  Donabedian model, x, 8, 9
  Health care Access and Quality Index (HAQ), 8–9
  and incentive alignment between patients, providers and payers, 41
  metrics for private-sector organizations, 65
  reducing iatrogenesis, 56

race, *see* ethnicity and race
remote patient monitoring (RPM), 85
rural areas
  and community providers, 157
  and health outcomes, 45
  and public–private partnerships (PPPs), 54
  and telehealth, 129
  as underserved, 40, 45–46

school-based health centers (SBHCs), 49
Singapore, 62, 124
social determinants of health (SDOH)
  CSDH conceptual framework, x, 103–105
  and health-related social needs (HRSN), 47–48
  as informing health care policy, x, 103, 105–107, 109–116, 117–118, 119, 122, 131–132, 142, 145
  integrating into health care delivery, 112
  introduction and overview, x, 1, 2–3, 107–108, 121–122
  as "medicine," 114–115
  structural vs. intermediary determinants of health, 105
  US Playbook, 111–112
  and the uninsured/under-insured, 32
social services, investment in, 112–113
South Africa, 110
South Korea, 62, *see also* Korea
Spain, 61, 124, 141
spending on health care. *see* costs and spending
substance use disorders, 80, 94, 140–141
Supplemental Nutrition Assistance Program (SNAP), 65
sustainability in health care policy, 130–131
Sustainable Development Goals (SDGs), 70
Sweden
  health care model and performance, 25, 62, 124, 131, 141
  integration of social determinants into health care policies, 131–132
Switzerland
  health care model, 35
  health care spending per capita, 26
  overall health care performance, 25, 62

Taiwan, 62
telehealth, 46, 48, 49–50, 61, 67, 82, 85, 129, 138, 142–143
Temporary Assistance for Needy Families (TANF), 65
Thailand, 111
transportation issues, 3, 47, 49, 121, 124
trust
  and active listening, 147
  and community-based care, 123, 124, 155, 157, 158, 164
  and depolarizing health care, 79
  and empathy, 146
  and health care workforce diversity, 141, 146
  and inclusive health care, 135
  and LGBTQ+-inclusive policies, 143
  and patient-centered care, 164
  and public–private partnerships (PPPs), 55
  reduced trust through partisanship and polarization, 72, 75–76
  and transparency, 65

underuse and unmet health care needs, 29, 42–43, 95, 125
uninsured/under-insured persons, *see also* Medicaid
   and ethnicity, 120, 121
   FQHC neighborhood clinics for, 49
   and lack of employer insurance coverage, 43
   limited impact of Affordable Care Act (ACA), 89, 92
   and mental illness, 32
   number of (US), 29, 32, 34, 121
   and unmet health care needs, 43, 121
United Kingdom
   health care model, 6, 35, 61, 118
   overall health care performance, 25, 26
   public vs. private health care service uptake, 60–61
   public–private partnerships (PPPs), 66
United Nations, Sustainable Development Goals (SDGs), 70
United Way, 66
universal health care
   benefits (overview), 125
   Beveridge model, xi, 5, 6, 61
   Bismarck model, xi, 5, 6–7, 61–62
   cost efficiencies, 125
   countries with, 29, 35, 124, 141, 150
   Essential Packages of Health Services (EPHS), 56
   funding models, 35, 50, 51, 150
   and international declarations and treaties, 70
   National Health Insurance Model, xi, 5, 7, 62
   as a political issue, 35, 38, 50–51, 70–71, 73–74
   and public–private partnerships (PPPs), 57–58
   resource requirements, 56
   role of data, 52
   as a Sustainable Development Goal (SDG), 70
upcoding (in health insurance), 97
urgent care clinics, 58, 61, 80, 82
utilization per person, and health care spending, 27–28

value-based models of care, 82
Veterans Health Administration (VHA), 6, 45, 71
virtual and augmented reality (VR and AR), 85

wait times
   and demand for services, 94–95
   and public vs. private health insurance, 51, 60
   and public–private partnerships (PPPs), 66
water quality, and health outcomes, 108
whole being model, x, 135–138, 147–148, 149–151
Women, Infants, and Children (WIC), 65
World Health Organization (WHO), 56
   Commission on Social Determinants of Health (CSDH), x, 103–105, 106
   early child development policies, 110–111
wrong pockets problem, 112

For EU product safety concerns, contact us at Calle de José Abascal, 56–1°,
28003 Madrid, Spain or eugpsr@cambridge.org.

www.ingramcontent.com/pod-product-compliance
Ingram Content Group UK Ltd.
Pitfield, Milton Keynes, MK11 3LW, UK
UKHW020409221225
466320UK00025B/1599